The Ultimate Guide
To A Multi-Orgasmic Life

by
Antonia Hall, MA

New Ventures Press
9663 Santa Monica Blvd., #1128
Beverly Hills, CA 90210
www.NewVenturesPress.com

Copyright © 2016 Antonia Hall

This publication is a creative work protected in full by all applicable copyright laws, as well as by misappropriation, trade secret, unfair competition, and other applicable laws. No part of this book may be reproduced or transmitted in any manner without written permission from New Ventures Press except in the case of brief quotations embodied in critical articles or reviews. All rights reserved.

The information, methods and techniques provided in this book are designed to provide helpful information to be used for self-improvement. This book is not meant to be used, nor should it be used, to diagnose or treat any medical condition. None of the information in this book is intended to replace appropriate medical and/or psychological treatment. The publisher and author are not responsible for any specific physical or mental health needs that may require medical supervision and are not liable for any damages or negative consequences from any treatment, action, or application to any person reading or following the information in this book.

First Edition, February 2016

Book cover design: Bill Greaves
Illustrations: Enrique "Kiki" Rosas
Author Photography: Nina Junger
Typesetting: Odyssey Books

Library of Congress Cataloging-in-Publication Data
Hall, Antonia.
The Ultimate Guide to a Multi-Orgasmic Life / Antonia Hall, MA.
1. Sex Instruction for men and women. 2. Sexual health. 3. Spiritual life. 4. Self-actualization (Psychology)—Religious aspects. I. Title.

Library of Congress Control Number: 2015959823
Paperback ISBN: 978-0-9970850-0-6
eBook ISBN: 978-0-9970850-1-3

Published in the United States of America

Dedication

This book is dedicated to all those seeking to bring more pleasure into their lives and to step into their greatest multi-orgasmic potential. By embracing and tapping into one's inherent sexuality, the positive benefits ripple outward into the world at large. I applaud your brave explorations into ways to honor yourself and your body, and wish you a meaningful, multi-orgasmic life that exceeds your wildest expectations.

Acknowledgements

I offer my deepest appreciation to those who have lent their support, guidance, and wisdom throughout the writing and publishing of this book. Thanks to Anna Emrey for her continual encouragement. I'm so grateful to Kathryn Hall for her sage counsel and for championing me on. Thank you to Bill Greaves for creating a beautiful cover, to Michelle Lovi for the gorgeous interior, to Enrique "Kiki" Rosas for the illustrations, and to Egan Hirvela for his gracious assistance. Jessica Gottlieb, Julia Kohn and Jason Fisher offered their kind observations and support. I'm appreciative for input from Richard Krawczyk, TJ Woodward, and publishers Marc Allen and Jessica Kristie. And, I give heartfelt gratitude to my cohort sisters and teachers, including Vicki Noble, Luisah Teish, D'vorah Grenn, Dianne Jenett and Marguerite Rigoglioso.

Contents

Dedication	iii
Acknowledgements	iv
Introduction	1
Section One: Mental Mastery	7
Documenting the Process	7
Opening to Ecstasy (Through the Resistance)	9
Know Thyself (It all Begins in your Mind)	13
The Path to Success	18
Hinderances: But I Have a Lot on My Mind	21
Creating What We Contemplate	24
Mindful Moderation	27
Heart Intelligence and Forgiveness	30
Be Grateful	32
Section Two: Essential Tools	37
Basic Grounding	37
Breath Awareness	40
Accessing Our Essence (Meditation)	44
Breath of Fire	46
Pelvic Bouncing	47
Tense and Release	49
Solar Lunar Breathing	50

Section Three: Playing with Energy   53
    Setting your Sexy Space   53
    Energy and What Science Already Understands   55
    Being Present   62
    How Energy Moves Throughout the Body   65
    What is Tantra and the Tao?   68
    Circulating Energy   71
    Circulating Energy for Another   73

Section Four: Physical Pursuits   75
    Anatomy   75
    Getting to Know Your Body More Intimately   84
    Fit is Sexy (and Feels Great)   86
    Why Yoga Matters   87
    Nourishment   90
    Stillness and Nature   92
    Types of Touch and Sweet Spots   94
    Sensory Experiences   98
    Toys and Lubricants   99
    Rhythms   105
    Soft-On Sex   107
    Positions for Success   109

Section Five: Orgasm Wisdom   113
    The PC Muscle   113
    Orgasms   118
    Benefits of Sex and Orgasms   124
    Full-Body Orgasms   127
    Becoming Multi-Orgasmic (For Men)   129
    Becoming Multi-Orgasmic (For Women)   134
    Kundalini   138

Section Six: Partnered Play   141
   Shakti and Shiva (Dance of the Feminine
    and Masculine)   141
   Intimacy   143
   Preparations   146
   The Art of the Kiss   148
   Reconnecting with Your Partner   150
   Asking for What You Want (and Having
    Your Needs Met)   153
   Keep Experimenting   157

About the Author   159

Introduction

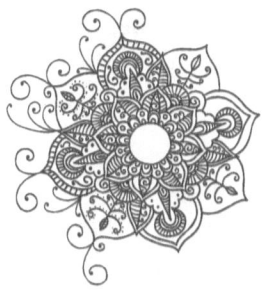

This book is a guide for both men and women on how to become multi-orgasmic and have mind-bending full-body orgasms. It's also a guide to finding fulfillment both in and out of the bedroom. I offer this book, dear reader, as a guide to ways that you can bring more pleasure, joy, creative flow and meaning into your life. Much of the information in this book was gathered during the last half of my life, which was further substantiated doing research for my Master's thesis. The more I incorporate into my daily life the techniques offered in this book, the happier and more fulfilled I feel on a day-to-day basis. While not all of the practices may immediately seem to relate directly to one's perceptions of sexuality, the techniques all enhance one's potential to live a richly fulfilling and multi-orgasmic life.

Sexuality is a natural part of human function. It's the fabric through which we were all created and part of being truly alive. Sexual energy is as natural and needed as the air we breathe or the food we need to nourish our bodies. Our bodies are not only wired for more pleasure than many people know is possible, but by tapping into this potent life force, it's possible for you to live an infinitely more joyful, flowing and happy life than you ever dreamed possible. Your energy will radiate outward into all areas of your life because sexual energy is creative, joyful, and fulfilling. Embracing and utilizing your innate sexual energy is a component of living your highest life potential.

Many of the techniques I describe in this book have been used successfully for thousands of years. Using the practices regularly can lend a centered revitalization throughout your everyday life. Each practice described is followed by an affirmation and a brief exercise to help you integrate the information. Each of the techniques I offer can be added to even the busiest of schedules, enriching your day. Once you've learned these practices, they can be a powerful and valuable resource you can draw upon for the rest of your life.

When I was in graduate school writing about and using these practices, I'd occasionally meet up with friends who hadn't seen me in some time, and they were always astounded when they saw me. They knew I'd been putting in a multitude of hundred hour weeks one after the next without a break and wanted to know how I was so energized, radiant, and happy. "It must be all of the full-body orgasms," I explained, with a smile on my face. It is my hope that you'll soon be able to say the same.

The Journey

In this book, I break up the teachings and techniques into a simple daily practice. The technique is detailed, then followed by an exercise, giving you a chance to implement the lesson. While some of these practices may not seem sexual, each is there to assist you with embracing the essential and highly creative sexual energy with which we were all born. These are practices I have found to be particularly life transforming. Many of the exercises I detail are centuries old. I hope to demystify esoteric language to bring these ancient teachings forth in a way that is relatable and easy to understand. I know from first-hand experience that these practices can allow for your sexual energy to be embodied in ways that lead to healing, growth and transformation, and that if you implement them, they'll infuse your life with a greater sense of trust, peacefulness and ecstatic joy. Most of these teachings are based upon and adapted from literature I have read through scholarly work and my own inquisitive nature, workshops I have attended, and personal experiences I have found to be valuable over decades. This is the book I wish I'd had when I first set out to learn Tantra and becoming multi-orgasmic. It is my hope that such offerings will inspire you to explore your sexuality in ways that empower and enrich your life.

Allow yourself to embark upon this new journey as an observer, noticing what feelings come up, but without placing judgements on it. Do you feel resistance to certain exercises? We all have different belief systems, influenced by how we were raised and the people we've continued to surround ourselves with, including media, entertainment and various institutions. If you experience a particular charge around views on sexuality, look at where this came from. Who taught you these rules on life, and are they working for you? Tune into what rings true for you. If you're willing to set aside limiting belief systems, you'll find this book full of tools that will transform your life. Hold the vision of yourself living a satisfying, multi-orgasmic life. Imagine yourself living life with more vibrant, joyous energy, your relationships being more loving and harmonious, and no longer being brought down and at the affect of outside influences. You will live from a place of your personal power and connection, have more creative energy, and experience attracting the people and experiences that support your life, rather than expending energy to chase things down, searching for something you feel is lacking in your life. You are creative, abundant and ripe to experience deep fulfillment. You may be having frequent mind-bending orgasms that roll through your whole body. That is what's meant by living a multi-orgasmic life. It is my wish that you step into your greatest multi-orgasmic life potential.

My Journey

To dare to tread where passion's pulse carries us
live fully, deeply within the moment
let heart's calling awaken
be nourished
and blossom.

—Antonia Hall

Sitting on a mat on the floor, I feel the firmness of the ground beneath me, letting my breath ground and connect me. My breath has been with me since the beginning, and will be with me until the end. Breath makes its way from my lungs into my bloodstream, exploring me from within, more deeply and more intimately than any lover could. A willingness to sit with my breath, expanding into it and its myriad shapes and possibilities, carries me into ecstatic states.

I was raised in a permissive household, post-Sixties freedom revolution. Sexuality and the naked body didn't come with shame attached. Curious about sexuality, I began reading up on and studying sexuality by my preteen years. Throughout my young adulthood I found myself in the role of teacher about sexuality and sexual reproduction for my peers.

In graduate school, I chose to complete my thesis studies contemplating the innate sexual energy of human beings, how this energy can be allowed healthy expression, and how this integration could improve our lives. I explored how psychologists and sexologists are encouraging women to embrace their sexual energy. I knew that by limiting ourselves by believing false narratives of sex as "sin," or that women are less libidinous, and with other shame-based thinking that can constrict our ability to express our true sexual nature, we limit our sense of self, authenticity, and potentials. I here exemplify methods through which humans for thousands of years have embraced their potent sexual energy, hopeful that it inspires readers to find a sense of vibrancy and passion in their own lives. Your potential is so great; I really hope you can make time and space, and find the courage to embrace your whole self fully.

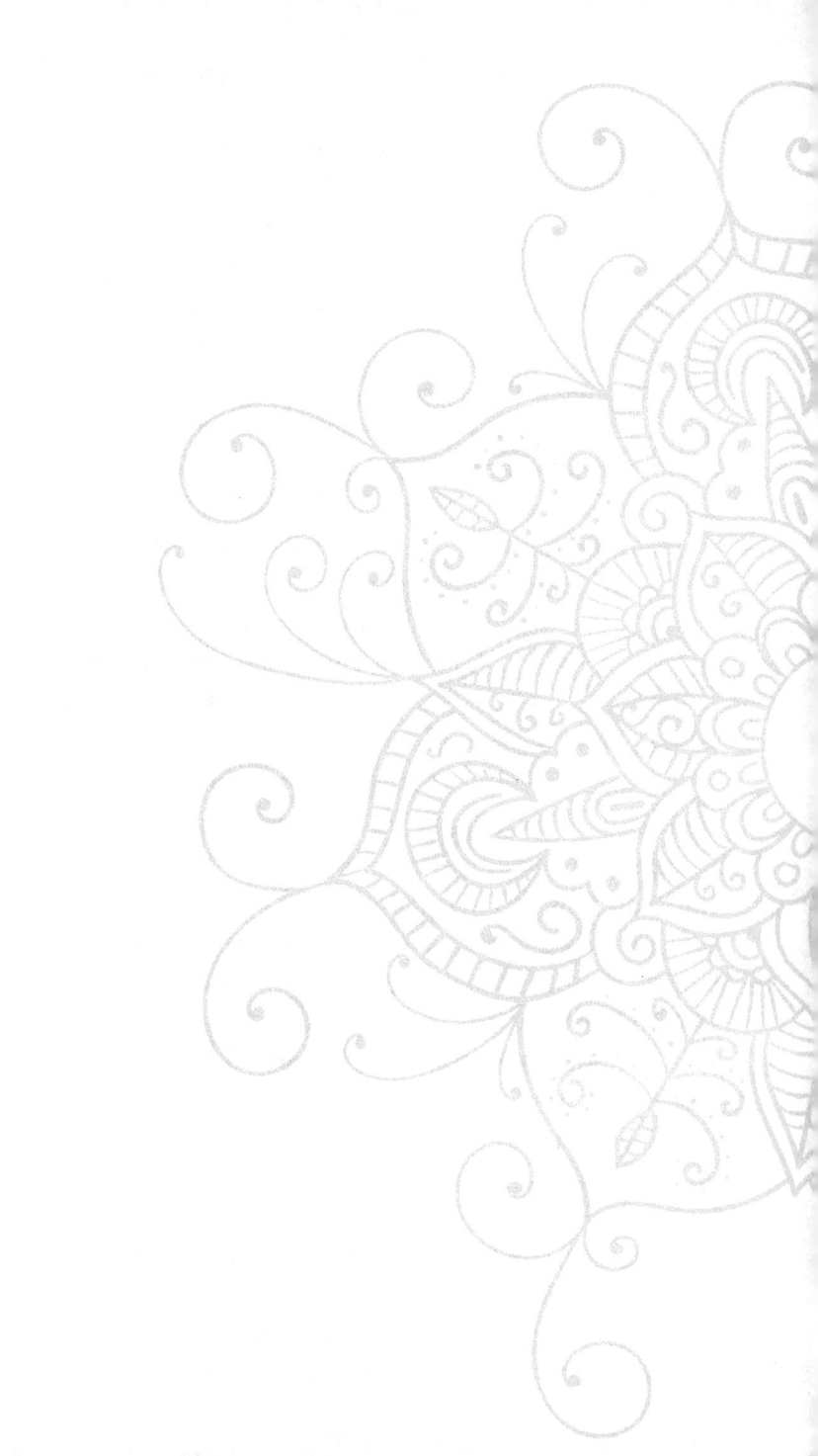

Section One: Mental Mastery

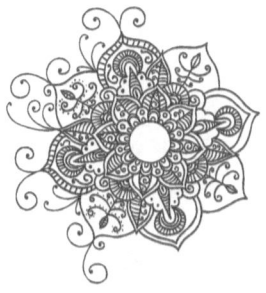

"When it comes to sex, the most important six inches are the ones between the ears."
—Dr. Ruth Westheimer

Documenting the Process

Keeping a journal can be an invaluable process. I write in my journal every morning, and find it to be an incredibly useful and worthwhile practice. I encourage you to invest at least a few minutes daily in writing in your own journal. From leather bound to black and white composition book, the journal itself can be as fancy or simple as you like. This is your own private place to document thoughts, emotions, fears, insights and breakthroughs. It's also a great place to document dreams, which can carry valuable information when we consciously choose to start listening to them.

Paint, draw, jot notes, or simply take pen to paper and rant. Writing in stream of consciousness form can provide wonderful revelations. Gain perspective by just letting thoughts flow through, without censorship or judgment. Give yourself permission to express in new and creative ways. Haikus, poetry or lists of words can impart clarity. Writing in my journal has served me with insights both in the moment and later when I re-read them. It has also resulted in increased creativity and receptivity. Everyone I know who journals finds it to be a worthwhile, helpful tool. While I know that adding one more thing to the 'to do' list may feel overwhelming, you'll actually be clearing thoughts from your mind, which will inevitably free you up. This is time just for you. It is an important and life changing journey to step into a multi-orgasmic life, one that will forever empower you. Journalling the process will greatly assist you in this worthwhile endeavor. I highly recommend you find the time of day that works best for you and give the gift of daily journaling to yourself.

Exercise: Let's get insightful! For the purpose of this incredible journey you're undertaking, get yourself a journal that best represents your commitment to living a multi-orgasmic life. Don't let finding the 'right' journal hinder you, but if you can find one that will remind you of your dedication to enriching your daily life and boldly stepping into your greatest potential, all the better. Begin by writing what you hope to accomplish through doing this program. Imagine yourself living your juiciest, most deliciously satisfying life. What does that look and feel like? How does that vibrancy infuse your everyday experience? Or, if this is too challenging at first, you may wish to write about how you ended up with the book, and the feelings that come up around the program. This is for you, and there are no right or wrong answers, only the willingness to explore.

Affirmation: I give myself permission to express myself in new and creative ways.

Opening to Ecstasy (Through the Resistance)

Just as with taking on any new activities, it's important to keep an open mind as you begin your explorations, and as you start learning the tools to live a multi-orgasmic life. Set aside expectations and approach it as an important expedition into ways you can enhance and enrich your life. Some of the techniques may be more familiar or comfortable, and others may bring up some feelings of resistance. We all have a history and story around our sexuality. I ask you to set the stories aside, and simply enjoy your sexuality. Freedom is a choice. Your body is wired to experience huge full-body orgasms that fuel you energetically. All you need are the tools to tap into it. Give this gift to yourself. I think you'll find this life changing.

This journey will require a commitment to setting

potentially limiting belief systems aside. Many of us were raised with messages that say that pleasure and sex are bad, dangerous, or sinful. These messages, which can come from family members, society, religion, or other outside sources, can become our own beliefs. But, pleasure and sex are basic biological, emotional and spiritual needs which enhance our health and well being. Sexuality needs expression as much as we need air, food, or water. By honoring this part of yourself in new ways, you'll learn how to step into a more powerful, creative version of yourself while expanding your capacity for pleasure and energizing other areas of your life. Without a willingness to look into and change our internal landscape, we cannot change our external world. Real growth asks that you step through your comfort zones, but this is a truly worthwhile venture.

While sex is a natural and innate part of being human, I believe that few of us in the Western World were raised with freedom to express this important and natural part of ourselves. Deep down many of us experience a vast discrepancy between what we're taught we should feel about sex and how we actually feel. Despite an intense sexual imagery reflected in our media and entertainment, I have heard many friends express their fears about embracing their sexuality. Mixed societal messages (such as the good girl/bad girl dichotomy) have created a vast discrepancy in our inherently sexual nature and our freedom to express it.

There are various reasons why one might shut themselves off from their sexual nature and the incredible potentials it holds. Statistics show that many people had negative experiences growing up, which may have included certain types of child and/or sexual abuse. Some people were raised with strict religious indoctrinations that taught them that sex is sinful and strictly for procreation. Perhaps a particularly hurtful relationship taught that it was safer to close off and not let people in. But through these constrictions, one only limits oneself and finds even greater discomfort. Often people will constrict themselves by closing off both physically and energetically. For many the physical restriction begins by limiting the breath, which limits what we can feel, including pleasure. Through breath and energy work, you can begin finding extended pleasure that will leave you energized for all other activities in your day. It is also a gateway to deep healing of past hurts and wounds, which are carried in the body and can hinder one's potentials for leading the happy, sexually fulfilled life we all deserve.

Are you ready to take back your own power and add more joyful creative energy into your life? Through looking at where difficulties may be holding you back, your life will forever be transformed. It's time to be bold, wild, creative and free. Throw away constructs like the good girl/bad girl or bad boy/good guy paradigms. You are part of Nature, which is inherently sexual. Your need for desire and pleasure is intrinsic, natural, healthy, and deserves to be expressed fully. Sexual energy is supposed to permeate our lives, just as it freely does in nature. It is not healthy to relegate sex to an act and to allow your sexual expression to be honored only on special occasions, or hidden away and turned inward. These limiting behaviors can lead to decreased awareness of the body and shortened orgasmic potentials rather than expanding them for increased pleasure. Your sexuality deserves daily attention, but in healthy ways that make you feel good about yourself, not shameful. Love your sexuality, and it will love you back in magnificent ways.

As you use the exercises in this book and begin to open your sexual energy through the Tantric-based practices I detail, notice feelings as they arise, but don't let fear paralyze you from expressing your most potent energy source. Anything newly ventured has a learning curve and requires moments of discomfort. Love yourself, and be compassionate with yourself during the process, and continue to acknowledge your own willingness to explore. Breathe through the resistance, fear, or worries that it isn't going to work. These are tried and true techniques which have carried many into ecstatic states for thousands of years. Are you ready to open yourself to your true potentials? If you don't do anything differently, your life will stagnate and stay the same. Acknowledge yourself for your willingness to try something new.

Life is too short to limit yourself, and when you embrace all parts of yourself, you can maximize your potentials and live the life of your dreams. Doing new things takes courage, and requires you to step outside of your comfort zones. Besides, this is play! Have fun with it. You're just learning to enjoy and appreciate your sexuality in new ways. The more you are willing to flex your sexually courageous muscles and play outside the box, the greater will be your capacity for experiencing vibrancy and an increased sense of passion in everyday life. This will allow for greater creativity, and increased success in all areas of your life.

Exercise: Get out your journal and answer these questions:
- What is your greatest fear about embracing your sexuality?
- In what ways will your life improve if you embrace your sexuality fully?

Affirmation: I embrace my sexuality and invite more pleasure into my life.

Know Thyself (It all Begins in your Mind)

It is time to explore the inner landscape. Like the ancient Greeks and Egyptian philosophers, Tantric texts speak to the importance of knowing thyself. What does that have to do with becoming multi-orgasmic and being sexually fulfilled? A lot! Pleasure derives from a mental place far more than it does down there. You need to know what's going on in that head of yours, which makes self-examination one of the first stages of stepping into a multi-orgasmic life.

Set your ego aside to examine who you are, what you believe, and why. Take time to admire the wonderful things about yourself, and also be honest about the impediments that may be getting in the way of living your fullest potential. How do you view the world around you? In Tantric philosophy, individuals are recognized as a piece of the cosmic whole of which we're all a part. Physics says that the universe is comprised of a unifying substance, just as Tantric texts have told us for thousands of years. Tantra says that the principle energy that created the universe resides within each of us, and by seeing yourself as a co-creator in this larger whole, you can open to amazing potentials of conscious manifesting. Scientific observation agrees that each portion of the universe contains the wholeness from which it was created. Tapping into this universal wholeness, moment by moment, allows you to stay in your greatest point of power. There's a natural flow to this, when you allow for it. I've found that the more I allow myself to be a part of this flow, the more my life unfolds with ease and grace. When I experience resistance and frustrations, I know that I am not trusting and flowing in the present moment.

In addition to staying in the present moment it is important to approach life and all you do with a loving positive attitude. This requires a shift in consciousness, but the more you learn to trust the dance of life and the experiences that are brought forth—even when they may appear to be challenges—the happier you'll be. Thoughts are a form of information-carrying energy, as modern science has proven. It is important to be mindful, rather than let old programming run unobstructed and unconsciously. Tantra refers to this positive approach in life as "the creative attitude," and it is related to the energy and visualization techniques used by professional athletes and successful business people. It may sound bogus, but by imagining yourself full of positive energy, for example, you stay in your power while creating a barrier to keep negative energies out. The ability to consciously keep your thoughts and attitude positive is an important part of psychological well-being. This journey asks you to make a commitment to self-love. As a part of your commitment to self-love, it is very important to bring greater awareness to your mindset.

Does your mind lead itself into positive thinking, or are you letting negative, fear-based programs operate? Are you able to watch your thoughts as though they were a crawl on CNN? The way our brains are able to quickly take in information, analyze it, and assess what we should do or say in a given moment is awesome. Truly. However, as the only thinker in your mind, it is up to you to be mindful and to change your own thinking and programming along the way. What old tapes are you letting run? Whether you're conscious of it or not, your thinking is affecting your everyday experiences of the world around you. Thoughts carry energy into the interconnected web of the universe, and returns mirrored back to us.

You don't always have a choice about challenges faced, but you can choose how you interpret these events. You surely know that interpretations have an affect on your mood, but you may not be aware of their consequences in your energy field. Pay attention to see if you are letting old mental tapes run, as you could be using your energy in an unproductive way, which in turn could be leading to lowered self-esteem, cynicism, pessimism, and negativity. Don't waste your energy getting caught up in the story of how it was, or how you fear it will be. You are in control and it is time to take back your power! The inner creates the outer.

As I eluded to, self-examination begins with observing your relationship to the things and events of the world. It's important to know what programming you carry. Whether it's an old program that tells you that you are not good enough, intelligent enough, or attractive enough, these old thoughts and belief systems will be reflected in the energy you put out into the world through your word and actions. This energy is then mirrored back to you by those around you and the universe at large.

Negative tapes can originate on the elementary school playground, the locker room after gym class, your home or work environment, or elsewhere. What's important is that you become aware of them and compassionately change them into positive thinking. Do you trust yourself? Or, have you been taught to acquiesce to the authority figures in your life, as is commonly taught? Do you live in a victim mentality, always complaining about the bad things happening to you? Are you often sick, or suffer from low energy? This can all stem from the old tapes you're allowing to play out in your mind, which in turn creates imbalances and blocks in your personal energy field. It's important to become aware of these patterns, and consciously change them.

How do you change your thinking from negative to positive? After bringing awareness to the voices to which you give energy, consciously rewrite them. Placing positive affirmations in plain view is a great way to begin this rewiring. Tape some affirmations to your bathroom mirror, refrigerator, car, and office. These affirmations are reminders that you are in control of your thoughts—and thoughts can be changed. Be aware. Watch your thoughts throughout the day, knowing that you are more than your brain, and in fact, you are the one in the driver's seat. Keep affirmations framed in the positive, present tense. "I am" statements are wonderful! "I am strong, beautiful, confident, smart, creative," etc. Fill in your "I am" statement for the areas in your life where you wish to consciously shift your thinking patterns. It is very powerful to write your own affirmations, and I would suggest you play with the messages you may need to reaffirm yourself.

Why do affirmations and changing your thought patterns from negative to positive thinking work? Because they reflect the truth. You are perfect just as you are. You came in that way. All else is egoic nonsense. Don't let old and outdated mental tapes control you and your life. You deserve the best, and it is time to allow the best into your life. Love yourself enough to become aware of what you are telling yourself and compassionately change the old, unhappy scripts into beautifully written, constructive ones. I will provide other practices later in this book to assist you with shifting into a healthier more enriching mindset, but the first step is to look at where you believe you are holding yourself back the most through negative mental programming.

Exercise: Make a list of five things you'd like to manifest for yourself. You may need to begin with the areas in your life you'd most like to change, then shift it into how this can be reinvented. So, if you're unhappy with your current job, make a statement of what you'd like to have instead. State it as though it's already come true in the form of a positive affirmation. Complete these affirmations for each of the five areas of your life you feel you most wish to change.

Affirmation: I practice bringing ever greater awareness to my thoughts.

The Path to Success

I wish to speak to the part of you that is clearly open to expanding into your true orgasmic potential. I want you to succeed, and this book offers every basic guideline, exercise and technique to get you there. However, sexuality has a way of wanting to open and blossom in its own sweet time, so I'm highly recommending that you let go of the outcome, and just thoroughly enjoy the process. We live in a goal-oriented society, and while wanting to step into your full sexual potential is a lofty intention, trying to make it happen could cause new resistances to arise. Just relax, enjoy yourself and trust that the process unfolds as it should. Orgasms happen when we are relaxed and surrendered, not goal focused. Spring always comes. Your multi-orgasmic abilities will too. Don't push or force, enjoy the deliciousness of the journey.

I know that the divide between where you are and where you wish to be can seem great. You can best bridge the two and succeed in these new endeavors by remembering that anything worth doing will take some time and determination. Grant yourself permission to take slow steady steps, and be realistic and compassionate with yourself throughout the journey, and you'll be far more likely to succeed. There will always be obstacles and excuses that you can use to keep you from moving forward with consistent determination, but if the process has true heart and meaning for you, it will be worthwhile to give it a resolute go. Here are some ways to assist you in arriving at the success you long for.

Hold the Vision – Spend a few minutes each day visualizing the success you wish to create for yourself. See yourself at the finish line of your goal. You've put in the work. What does your multi-orgasmic life look and feel like? Referring back to your journal notes is an excellent way to stay in touch with your desired outcome.

Take a New Step Each Day – Take one action toward the goal each and every day. Even the smallest step is movement in the right direction. Each of these chapters is short and easy to implement into even the busiest schedule. The more advancements you make, the better you'll feel, and the closer you'll be to fulfilling your multi-orgasmic dreams. Taking these practices in manageable increments will lead to big results.

Quiet the Naysayers – Naysaying can arrive through well-meaning loved ones, friends, or our own internal voices. Often times it is our own inner critic that can be our biggest challenge. What fears are holding you back? Are you more afraid of failure or success? Do you fear the intensity of deep sexual fulfillment? Stand up for yourself, and your right to experience the pleasure we are all wired for. You don't have to tell anyone that you're undertaking this journey. Write about it in your journal, and only share when it feels appropriate.

Want it More – You have to want to honor your sexuality. The body is wired to have huge mind-blowing full-body orgasms. Are you willing to put in the effort? Want it more than the urge to check your social media stream, peruse the internet, or space out in front of the television. Distractions will present themselves, especially when you've made a commitment. The trial lies in continuing the journey despite them.

Enjoy it to the Fullest – Remember why you wanted to do this. If your heart and body longed for embracing your sexuality in new ways and fulfilling orgasmic potential you've wondered if you were capable of, then the process will be juicy, delicious and fun! Enjoy each step in the journey to the fullest. And, keep breathing. Breathe is the key.

Exercise: Take out your journal and answer these questions:
- What is your greatest resistance to learning to be multi-orgasmic?
- What would you gain by releasing this resistance and continuing with the journey?

Affirmation: I joyfully welcome a multi-orgasmic life.

Hinderances: But I Have a Lot on My Mind

Men and women can experience roadblocks to having an orgasm. Let's look at some of the most common reasons. In order to experience sexual release of orgasm, we must find a balance of a physical awareness, with a psychological and energetic mindfulness. Sometimes there are underlying issues within ourselves or the relationship we're in that might prevent our ability to surrender to sexual openness. Are there issues in your relationship? Are you tired or overly stressed? Are you harboring feelings of guilt or shame? Or are you experiencing an honest lack of sexual desire? Once you can get in touch with the underlying block, you'll have the ability to release it. By letting go and learning to relax, your energy will flow and you'll expand your ability to experience sexual fulfillment.

In order for orgasm to occur, the body needs to be able to have healthy blood flow and nerve supply. Anything from disease, illnesses, medications, being severely out of shape, or excessive drinking or drug use can decrease arousal and orgasmic potential. Some common medications for high blood pressure, depression, and pain can all lead to reduced sex drive, the ability to become aroused, or ability to reach orgasm. Speak with your doctor about lowering dosages or switching your medications, if this is the case.

Women who have had genital or pelvic surgery may also experience difficulty with blood flow or lubrication necessary for proper arousal. There is promising evidence that through healthier lifestyle choices, these can be improved. We will look at some of these in later chapters, but avoid smoking, eat a balanced diet, exercise and find self-loving ways to reduce the stress and anxiety in your life. The use of the energy exercises can also greatly improve these conditions, releasing blockages brought about by trauma, fear or other painful experiences.

When there are relationship challenges, it is difficult for couples to continue being intimate. Intimacy and finding orgasmic pleasure together requires openness, trust and the ability to relax with each other. I will detail exercises to enhance intimacy later. Remember that your partner is your best friend. Be honest, but kind and compassionate in the way you communicate. Interestingly, the more you begin utilizing the exercises to find compassion and self-love, the more this will ripple out into your connection with your partner.

For various reasons, there is commonly a time in many men's lives when they experience difficulty getting an erection or ejaculating far more quickly than they would like. While this can seem like a serious wound to the ego and one's sense of manhood, it is pretty common and one should never assume that it's permanent. Different times in our life can bring stressors or low energy levels that contribute to this situation, and there is a danger that these often temporary difficulties can become internalized. This can lead to fear-shame cycles, which perpetuate the situation. The ability to get an erection is also linked directly to how a man is feeling about himself, so if life has been challenging, this can easily lead to one's decreased desire. Also note that gravity draws blood away from the penis when a man is on his back, so try shifting positions to see if this is helpful in getting and maintaining an erection.

The Tantric philosophy perceives ejaculating sooner than you or your partner would like to be unnecessary and preventable. Through learning your arousal cycle and how to postpone ejaculation you can take your power back. Being able to stop before the point of no return is essential, as well as learning to move energy away from the sex organs. All of this is detailed in upcoming chapters. The breathing exercises and meditation practice can assist in producing a calmer, more relaxed outlook, which helps with moving through any undesired sexual hindrances.

If it has been some time since you've been able to get an erection, test to ensure that there is no physiological reason. Men have at least one or two erections at night. Lick a strip of postage stamps and attach them in a ring around your penis before going to sleep. If the ring is torn when you awaken in the morning, you are able to get an erection. Look at other factors which could be contributing, such as diabetes, back issues or spinal cord injuries, antidepressant usage or other medications, alcoholism, or hardening of the arteries. You may want to seek professional assistance if has become a continued challenge.

Exercise: Be honest with yourself. Get out your journal and write about hinderances you feel could be getting in the way of your leading a fulfilling multi-orgasmic sex life. Are you using a busy schedule as an excuse? Are you avoiding issues with your partner, or are there other unhealthy habits that could be getting in the way? Being willing to admit and address blocks is necessary in order to get past it. Know that you are worthy of leading the happiest, most satisfying and healthy life possible.

Affirmation: I release my limitations and open to the ecstasy of life.

Creating What We Contemplate

Many of the great intellectual minds of our recent and distant past have touted the importance of using our imagination to create our reality. As scientific data indicate, our future is not out there in a set form, we create it as we go along. Now, if you continue to live your life believing only in ordinary everyday reality or within limited constructs of your own power, you can expect few changes in your life. But, life allows us to use tools to grow, expand, and create anew. Using the power of your imagination is one of the most potent tools upon which you can rely to consciously create and manifest the life you dream of and desire. We tend to unlearn how to use our imaginations as we move from childhood to adulthood, but like any muscle, you can begin to strengthen this skill through practice.

The power of imagination has many practical applications. Top athletes pay coaches to help them visualize their successes so they can reach their physical goals and surpass their prior successes. Business managers and sales people have used visualization techniques to help them meet their target objectives. Writers, artists, philosophers and even scientists rely on their natural propensity for creative imaginations to aid their projects. One needs a vast inner landscape to discover new worlds.

The brain continuously reprograms itself through images. Science shows that we have the ability to imprint our own wishes into the physical universe around us and physics tells us that focus changes outcomes that would otherwise remain the same. Using your imagination every day will help you improve your life, including your sex life. Remember how energy flows with our intention and awareness? All is energy.

Learning to switch off the mental chatter is a valuable skill. The sexual secrets flourish when put to use in the creative mind. Using your imagination can allow you to move from feelings of stress to inner calm. It increases your creative drive, and is a great tool for modeling your world. Plus, it's just fun. Play like when you were a child. Turn off the inner dialogue and relearn to foster your imagination. It will allow you to kindle your sexual potentials and will strengthen your ability to manifest the life you desire.

Exercise: Train your imagination every day. I recommended earlier in this book that you make a commitment to visualizing your success each day. I'd still love for you to do that, but I'm now also inviting you to spend at least five minutes each day closing your eyes and expanding your imaginative powers. From this day forward, you will consciously spend time using your imagination as the conscious creational tool that it is. Close your eyes and see yourself within the outcome you desire to achieve. It would be wonderful if you imagined yourself living in your full multi-orgasmic potential and place of power. Stay focused on the desired vision, letting all other thoughts to be transitory, coming back to the goal. Focus upon the details of your outcome, challenging yourself to bring more and more detail to it as the days and weeks progress.

Remember that your imagination is not just a picture on a screen. It should include as much rich detail as possible. Use all of your senses to bring your interior world to life. One way to step into this world is to envision a building. Build on it each day in your mind's eye. Feel the ground beneath your feet. How does the light hit the floor, walls, and shine through the windows? Imagine every detail using all of your senses and really step into the vision to the best of your ability. Live it in your mind. Listen for the sounds there. Are there birds? People? What can you hear? What does it smell like? Are there pine trees? Hibiscus flowers? Perhaps a hint of jasmine wafts through on the breeze, passing through the open window. What physical sensations can you experience? Can you feel the air gently caressing your skin? What feelings or emotions do these evoke? Make it playful and fun for yourself. This is your world. You can imagine your future home, or a candy world with butterscotch rivers and marshmallow chairs, if you desire. Get creative!

Affirmation: With the wonder of a child, I open to my creativity and imagination.

Mindful Moderation

Everything is an opportunity for learning and growth. In Tantric philosophy there is no judgement around sexual preferences, nor are certain sexual acts deemed acceptable or unacceptable. All explorations are seen as an opportunity to become more of who we are and integrate various parts of ourselves. However, this does not mean that one should not practice discernment. Self-indulgence is not recommended and shows a lack of emotional maturity. Doing things which harms oneself or another's well being is indicative of a psychological or emotional imbalance. In Western culture, numbing out as a method of coping is commonplace, and well accepted. This does not make it healthy. Nor will it allow you to step into your greatest potential and life purpose. Moderation is key in everything.

It is important to be honest with oneself about one's behavior patterns. Are you doing something because it is worthy of your time and attention? Or, is it distracting you from something you don't want to be thinking about or doing? Suffering is unavoidable in life, but letting the hurt and negative feelings remain only increases your suffering. Until we face and let go of old hurts, we carry them with us, letting them cast a shadow on our perceptions and lives. They can influence our expectations, and burden us with internal doubts and fears.

Many people cope with their fears and hurts by dulling, denying, avoiding, and/or suppressing them. Numbing with addictions such as food, alcohol, or drugs, is an avoidance strategy that begins and ends with fear and lack of self-love. One cannot outrun oneself. It will only perpetuate feelings of inadequacy, shame, futility and guilt. I know life can bring some painful challenges, but covering up hurts and pretending we're not in pain doesn't work for anyone. Are you using unhealthy coping mechanisms? Be honest about whether it's something you can get through on your own, or if you need assistance from a professional.

If you have been using pain-avoidance practices, identifying them is the first step in releasing them. Then you get to make a more conscious choice next time you use them. Have these habits really helped to make life better, happier, or healthier? Admit to yourself that you are hurting or are suppressing fears you haven't wanted to face. What was the cause? How long do want to give your power away to it? You have the ability to change this. You deserve to live a fulfilling life, which is accessible once you've freed yourself from self-limitations. The more we suppress our pain, the more we numb out the ability to experience pleasure, too.

Could there be better balance and moderation in your life? Do you need to apologize to yourself or others? In the next chapter we'll explore the power of forgiveness, which should never be underestimated. Life is too short to carry these burdens and allow them to limit your precious potential. You have gifts to bring forth in the world, and addictive patterns and dwelling in the past will limit and restrict you, while the fear, pain, and hurt remain through the numbness. These negative patterns also make it very challenging to ever live your greatest potential or a multi-orgasmic life.

Exercise: In your journal reflect upon the questions posed, and be honest about what coping mechanisms you may be using to numb out your hurts. How are these pain-avoidance techniques showing up in your life, and how are they affecting your relationship with yourself and others in your life? Are there changes that need to be made? Can you do it alone, or do you need to get some assistance? The breath and energy work in this book are powerful tools for healing, but be honest about whether or not you can release addictive and unhealthy habits alone. You deserve to live the most amazing, fulfilling life; don't let hurts from the past take that away from you.

Affirmation: I maintain a healthy balance by treating myself with love and respect.

Heart Intelligence and Forgiveness

The heart is a powerful healer. It has a 'brain' all its own. There is a lot of research that has been going into heart intelligence and the powerful way that tapping into our heart energy can bring about transformations in the way we relate to others and the world around us. Humans are wired to want to share love, the essence of our being, with others. The more we close this area off by holding onto anger, frustrations, resentments and disappointments, the less we are able to love ourselves and others. It also limits the capacity and ability to experience ecstasy. This, in turn, reduces our ability to let the heart and brain work synergistically.

We've all experienced some form of hurts in our lives, and until we can find forgiveness, these hurts become blocks that hinder our ability to live fully and happily. Forgiveness is not about the person, people or situation you deem to have wronged you. It is about yourself, as ultimately it is a gift to yourself. Through finding forgiveness, you will free yourself from the pain and weight you otherwise carry with you into your relationships with others and attitude toward life. When we carry unresolved anger and frustrations, we aren't getting even with someone or something that hurt us, we are damaging ourselves. These old wounds are the bitterness that poison your life day to day, and keep you in an endless cycle destined to repeat these same patterns of pain and disappointment. You deserve better. I know it's not always easy to let go, but I urge you not to let the past prevent you from living your best life. Forgive in order to allow for your own healing, growth and happiness.

You can begin the healing process by accepting the situation. There are some really horrific situations that can arise in life, but it is essential to make peace with the past so you can begin to live your future. Dwelling on and reliving these hurts doesn't serve you or your well being. Recognize that you're the one in control, and take your power back by making a commitment to moving forward through forgiveness. It takes real strength to make peace with the past and forgive the situation and those involved.

If you are truly desiring to become multi-orgasmic and add full body orgasms to your repertoire, you'll need to also find forgiveness and make peace with your past. Don't carry the stories around with you as armor. These just lead to perpetual patterns of victim mentality, whereby you're getting attention from others by way of pity. This only limits you and your potentials. Let go. Go to the mirror, look yourself in the eyes and tell yourself, "I Love you." Yes, out loud. Say it daily, or every time you see yourself in the mirror. At least three times per day. Bow to your beauty. Honor your limitless potential. Find forgiveness and know that you are worthy of it.

It's important to honor the processes, and feel your feelings. But don't cling to the wounds. Holding onto or dragging wounds with you for years is unhealthy. You'll only diminishing your own life. Let go, and free yourself to move on to new, more joyful experiences.

Exercise: Think of someone in your life you'd like to forgive. Look at the lessons you've learned from this experience. Breathe love and forgiveness into the story. Forgive them and set yourself and them free. Journal your feelings about this experience, and how forgiving will allow you to move on. Are you willing to release the wound so you can recreate stories from a place of strength and your own power? Or are you determined to hold onto it so you can relive that wound over and over again? You are loved. You deserve to be loved. Do you know this at the core of your being?

Affirmation: I release past hurts by forgiving myself and others.

Be Grateful

The next mental tool we're going to explore is the power of gratitude. I know that gratitude may seem like quite the departure from having multiple orgasms, but orgasms are far more connected with your state of mind than your sex organs. It has been my experience that by staying in a state of gratitude your life will begin to transform in incredible ways. There are many scientific studies that indicate that choosing to put one's focus on gratitude increases feelings of happiness. Thoughts of gratitude stimulate the hypothalamus, which is a key part of the brain in stress regulation. Grateful thinking can also stimulate the ventral tegmental area of the brain, which leads to pleasurable sensations. Effects of gratitude can not only transform one's life, but also allows for better relationships with others. The more you can embrace life and the people in it with a creative and grateful attitude, the more you learn to trust yourself and the universe.

Begin with an intention to consciously move your thoughts away from what's not working to things for which you can be grateful. We are all comprised of conscious energy in motion. When your energy focus shifts from what you don't want in your life to what you want more of, you will begin to feel an attitude change, both internally (where everything begins) and externally (which is a reflection of the inner). This shift changes how you relate with the outside world. Embrace gratitude every chance possible and you'll find that more gifts will be brought into your life. Additionally, you'll find it easier to stay in the present moment, which is where your true power resides. Rather than giving your potent life energy to concerns with how things were in the past, or worrying about what may happen in the future, you can show up in the moment as a fuller version of yourself.

If you're not already accustomed to embracing an intention of gratitude in your life, I would recommend beginning a gratitude journal. Writing things down is a great resource and powerful practice. You may choose to use the journal you started at the beginning of this process, but I would encourage beginning a gratitude journal that is exclusively for the practice of extending your thanks to the universe for all of the blessings it's gifting into your life. Find a comfortable, quiet place to sit undisturbed. Reflect upon the different areas of your life, making note of the things for which you are genuinely grateful. If the emotion is not there, the result will reflect this, so choose that which resonates a true emotional feeling of gratefulness. Make a commitment to yourself that you will do this at least once per day. It doesn't take very long, but it will make a big impact on your life. Even five minutes a day is better than not doing it at all. Put in the time you can spare for awhile and notice how it starts to change your thinking, and how this gets carried throughout your day.

Eventually your need for a gratitude journal will be replaced by a consistent and genuine attitude of gratitude. An awareness will seep into your consciousness that good things are happening on a day-to-day basis. By letting go of fears and worry thinking, you'll trust that everything is working toward your highest good. Your resistance to challenges melts away, and you'll be able to remind yourself that while what's going on that would normally cause stress and upset may not be meeting your pictures, it will bring its own rewards. For example, a stranger hit my car the first day I moved to San Francisco. My car was an older car, which had been with me for many years and wasn't worth much, but it still ran well and I was sentimental about keeping it. I was understandably upset when I returned to the parking lot where I'd left my car and saw that it was smashed up. But then I surrendered, and shifted to a place of trust that it was in my best interest. Sure enough, the insurance company cut me a decent sized cheque. It may not have met my pictures, but it was a gift in the end.

There is a Native American saying, "Give thanks for unknown blessings already on their way." By writing in a gratitude journal each day, you're well on your way to learning this potent manifestation tool.

Exercise: Start a gratitude list. Challenge yourself by starting with the basics, then expanding out to everything in your life for which you can be grateful. Continue the practice until it becomes second nature.

Affirmation: I express my gratitude and my life flourishes.

Section Two: Essential Tools

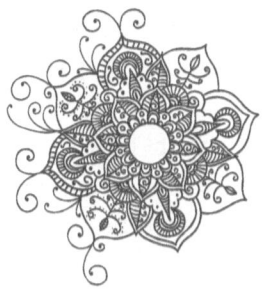

"Your task is not to seek for love, but merely to seek and find all the barriers within yourself that you have built against it."
—Jalāl ad-Dīn Muhammad Rūmī

Basic Grounding

The first physical practice I'm introducing is a basic grounding exercise, as I want you to use it before any other practice you use in this book. If you're not familiar with grounding the body, I think you'll appreciate what using it each morning will bring to your day. It's very simple to do and it lends a greater sense of stability and peace as you go about your daily tasks. When you are grounded, you are not as likely to be thrown off balance by surprises or stressors that come your way. It provides an anchor to assist you with staying in the present moment while you go about activities, so you're less likely to be thrown off balance or feel frazzled.

While there are various ways to ground energy, there are some basic principles I've found to be important. If you've never used grounding techniques before, you'll want to begin by bringing awareness into your physical body. My favorite visualization for grounding is to imagine becoming like a great rooted tree. Once you become more familiar and comfortable with this practice, you'll be able to do it quickly in various environments, and even simultaneously with other activities. I'll also be building upon this exercise as we progress further into multi-orgasmic living practices.

Exercise: Get comfortable, sitting or standing, spine straight, with your feet flat on the floor. Bring awareness to your breath, which should be natural, and not forced. As you inhale, relax your belly and allow air to flow into your body as a result of this expansion of the abdomen. Allow your attention to turn inward. You may want to put your hand on your belly to bring awareness there, as you continue to breathe. There are three parts to the breath: the inhale, the retention and the exhale. As you inhale, you are bringing life-giving energy into your body. During retention those energies can be consciously extracted and circulated throughout the body. With your exhale, imagine releasing any tension and negativity you may have accumulated in your body. Visualize your body filling with breath, all the way to your fingertips, the top of the head and down to your toes.

Bring your awareness to your tailbone or the base of your spine. Imagine a thick cord running from this point all the way to the center of the earth. With each breath (I like to do this on the exhale, but do what feels right to you) picture this cord becoming brighter and thicker as it makes its way through the soil, rocks, deep into the core of the earth. Once you feel deeply rooted into the center of the earth, ensure that you have a good connection. You are now grounded.

If using grounding exercises is new to you, you should practice the basic method above everyday for a week before moving on to the extended charging energy exercise I detail next. This exercise can take a few minutes or longer, depending upon what feels needed and comfortable to you. This is an easy one to implement into your life. It can be done in the shower each morning, or before you get out of bed. When you first awaken, stretch, come into your body and ground yourself. Having a grounding chord throughout the day will help keep you in the present moment. Make it a daily routine to ground early in the day, and again throughout the day, as needed. You'll also use this grounding exercise prior to any breathing techniques, energy work and the powerful sexual practices I detail later.

Affirmation: I am centered and balanced as I go about my day.

Breath Awareness

One of the most powerful tools one can use is breath. It's easy to carry on with life without thinking about having to breathe, but automatic breathing is oftentimes shallow. Through consciously tuning into the air as it makes its way into your lungs, expanding your body, you connect with your physical form, nourishing yourself internally. A few deep breaths taken consciously throughout the day can dispel stuck energies, energizing and uplifting you. Once I learned these techniques, I found that breathwork alone could bring about ecstatic states.

Breathwork is also an important concept in Tantra, where the saying "breath is life" speaks to this vital tool. In order to lead a multi-orgasmic life, you must be able to experience yourself from within, and breath is the vehicle that can take you there. Breath connects you with your creative sexual energy and amplifies physical sensations. You're also going to learn to move energy throughout your body with breath. It's very difficult to experience deep pleasure without breathing into it. It is such a powerful tool, which is why this chapter is so close to the beginning. Please gift yourself with daily breathwork (like the exercises below), so you can learn to relax and expand into multi-orgasmic living.

By taking shallow breaths, you will actually feel "less," which can become an unhealthy, escapist coping technique. You may be thinking that you already know how to breathe. It is something that occurs to us automatically, spontaneously, and naturally. You are able to breathe without thinking about it consciously, so it may seem foolish to think that you can be told how to breathe.

Yet, one's breathing becomes modified and restricted in various ways, not just momentarily, but habitually. One can develop unhealthy habits without being aware of it, such as slouching, which diminishes lung capacities and leads to chronic shortened breaths.

Most of us breathe by expanding our chests, using our upper back and neck muscles to raise the rib cage. Our breathing is too shallow and too quick. We are not taking in sufficient oxygen and we are not eliminating sufficient carbon dioxide. As a result, our bodies are oxygen starved, and a toxic build-up occurs. Every cell in the body requires oxygen and our level of vitality is just a product of the health of all the cells. This leads to increased disease. Our resistance to disease is reduced, since oxygen is essential for healthy cells. This means we catch more colds and develop other ailments more easily. Lack of sufficient oxygen to the cells is a major contributing factor in cancer, heart disease, and stroke.

Conscious breathwork is one of the fundamental tools for healthier living and a multi-orgasmic life. Connecting with your inner self at this level can also lead to powerful transformations and potent ecstatic experiences. Additionally, by utilizing breathwork exercises and consciously breathing throughout the day, you will increase vital energy in your body. Life-expectancy is linked to the frequency of breathing in the Yogic traditions. Explore, allow, expand into breath, letting the air nourish you more deeply and intimately than any lover could. Through continued breathwork, you may easily find that deep breathing allows for ecstatic states and may even lead to some pretty amazing orgasms.

Exercise: Below you will find three different breathing techniques to enhance your energy levels and multi-orgasmic potential. Become familiar with each of these breathing techniques and begin incorporating them into your daily life. Find which ones contribute to helping you destress, relax, energize, or uplift. The more tools you have in the toolbox to rely upon the better.

Basic Nourishing Breath – One of the basic breathing techniques found in Tantric practices is a basic nourishing breath. If you're new to conscious breathwork, begin by lying on your back. Otherwise, sit comfortably with a straight spine. Begin by yawning and opening the back of your throat. Let your mouth fall open and breathe gently and fully. Don't force the air in or out, just let your exhale release in a gentle sigh. Keep your throat open so you can take in as much air as you can in an effortless way. Keep breathing for about three to five minutes. This simple but powerful breath can be used to expand into the body during the day, and also during sexual activity.

Healing Breath – Get comfortable lying on your back. Place your left hand on your heart and right hand on your belly. Close your eyes. You'll be breathing through your nose for this exercise, so you may want to close your mouth, as well. Take a deep breath through your nose, sending the air into your belly. Feel the rise in your right hand as the belly fills, holding the breath for a count of four. As your exhale (through your nose), focus on the air leaving first your belly, then the lungs. This may feel strange if you've been a shallow breather for some time. Continue for five to ten minutes.

The Healing Breath will teach your body to breathe more deeply, which also lowers heart rate. This breathing technique is especially useful to men so they can master practices described later on.

Smile Your Way to Bliss Breath – Regardless of how you're feeling, you really can trick your body by smiling your way to bliss. I know that "putting on a happy face" may seem artificial. But, it's actually easy to trick the body by allowing a genuine smile to spread through your body, creating a powerful sense of relaxation. It is a subtle change in facial expression, a half-smile, which should extend through your eyes and the corners of your mouth. Smile both outwardly and inwardly, allowing the smile to spread throughout the body, letting tension release. You want to capture the feeling of "ahhhhhhh...," relaxation. If you can't do it, try forcing a big belly laugh ("ha-ha-ha"). That will get you to smile! Sexual ecstasy comes from a place of relaxation, so completing these exercises at least once a day will really contribute to your multi-orgasmic attainment.

Lie down on your back and close your eyes. Place a hand on your stomach, and the other on your chest. Relax the back of your throat and jaw, and take a good gentle breath. If you're like most people, your chest expands but your stomach doesn't move much. This will change as you utilize these breathing exercises more often.

Most people naturally breathe through their stomach in this position. Take a few normal breaths to be sure your stomach expands as you inhale, and contracts as you exhale. Once you have the hang of it, continue breathing this way. You may place your hands wherever they feel most comfortable. Now, let that semi-smile spread from your lips and eyes and allow the energy to spread through your body. As your thoughts wander and your smile fades, just bring yourself back to an awareness of your breath and smile. Once you are blissfully relaxed, open your eyes, but continue to sit with the sensation of your breath and the smile. When ready, sit up, but continue to breathe from your stomach. And remember to smile.

Affirmation: I find expansion and pleasure through awareness of my breath.

Accessing Our Essence (Meditation)

Even knowing and having experienced the benefits of meditation, there are times when I don't want to take the ten to twenty minutes per day to do it. Then I remind myself of the immense benefits. Do you have a meditation practice already? Have you always meant to get to it? Now would be a really good time to make that commitment. Tantra teaches that meditation is a powerful tool for getting to know yourself, and recent research is confirming the multitude of benefits. Meditation stills the mind and the tapes that play there, helping you access the essence of your being. This clarity will carry through into your everyday life, allowing you to stay more harmonious. I found it particularly helpful when I lived in chaotic Los Angeles, and while I was in graduate school. In the end, you'll realize, as I did, that meditation is worthwhile regardless of your current life story or situations. It can also assist with increasing your capacity for pleasure.

There is an old zen adage that says, "You should sit in meditation for twenty minutes every day—unless you're too busy; then you should sit for an hour."

There are numerous benefits to meditation. You will feel calmer, less reactive and more balanced as you go about your daily life tasks. Your interactions with others will become more harmonious. You will feel happier, less stressed and have a greater sense of inner peace, as well as an increased knowledge of who you are. There are also numerous health benefits to having a daily meditation practice. Did I mention decreased stress, depression and anxiety? This is because meditation shifts brain activity from the stress-prone right frontal cortex to the calmer left frontal cortex. This in turn decreases brain activity in the amygdale, which is where the brain processes fear. This leads to better concentration, increased blood flow, lower blood pressure, decreased muscle tension, increased serotonin production, enhanced immune system function, reduced symptoms of premenstrual syndrome, and better sleep. All in just ten to twenty minutes per day!

There are many methods of meditation, so explore various methods to find those that work best for you. You may find that you enjoy using a concentration method, by which you can use an external object to focus and anchor yourself into the present moment. For example, a lit candle flame can provide a focal point for such a practice. Another good one for beginners is to sit or lie down (just keep your spine straight) and focus upon your breath as it makes its way in and out of your lungs. This is a version of "mindfulness" meditation whereby you mindfully allow thoughts to flow through, without allowing any one of them to gain your real focus. Rather, you stay focused on your breath.

Exercise: Choose a method of meditation you feel will work best for you and begin practicing daily. Begin with ten minutes per meditation period. If you are already meditating daily, challenge yourself to find new forms or deepen your practice. Afterward, take notes in your journal to record your experiences.

Affirmation: I feel calm, peaceful and grounded.

Breath of Fire

This is a powerful Tantric breathing exercise to increase fire energy and revitalize your body known as the Breath of Fire. This breathing technique spreads heat throughout the body, and is very energizing.

Breath of Fire Exercise: Done while sitting or standing, spine straight, the Breath of Fire is a continuous breathing technique done entirely through the nose with an emphasis on the exhale. As you exhale, push air out of your nostrils while pulling your navel toward the spine. Release your belly outward, letting your lungs fill with air. To start, breath every two seconds, then working up to one to two breaths per second. Practice for no more than one to two minutes. Charge and energize your body with this powerful breathing practice.

Affirmation: My breathe cleanses and energizes me.

Pelvic Bouncing

Sometimes energy seems to stagnate around the lower part of the body. This may be experienced as a build up you're unaccustomed to as you begin to cultivate your sexual energy. Or, perhaps you would just like another new pleasurable way to move energy and have full-body orgasms. I love this one, and use it most mornings after a warm shower, before beginning the day. You'll feel more alive, connected, and may also experience intense pleasure as you use these exercises. Additionally, you'll learn to understand that your body is a gateway to divinity and that sexuality is one of the easiest and most profound ways to access this connection. For now, play and have fun with it.

Please remember to use a grounding technique prior to doing this exercise.

Pelvic Bouncing Exercise: To begin the bouncing pelvis exercise, lie flat on your back on a yoga mat, thick quilt, or well-carpeted area. It's important to have enough padding so you do not hurt your lower back area while you're bouncing. Bend your knees keeping your feet fat on the floor hips width apart, heels comfortably close to your buttocks. Stretch your neck. Open your mouth wide once to open the throat, then relax your jaw. Start bouncing your pelvis off of the ground, beginning slowly and gently then increasing the speed. Find a rhythm that is comfortable for you. It may feel like work in the beginning, but don't give up. You should feel your energy move up your spine, and you may want to visualize this as golden light. As energy moves, the body can quiver or shake, and emotions stored in these energy centers may arise. Breathe and release, expanding into this nurturing energy.

You may also choose to circulate the energy you raise. Remember to keep the tip of your tongue at the back of your front top teeth and bring breathe and awareness to the energy's movement. Yum!

Affirmation: My energy is flowing and I feel alive and connected.

Tense and Release

Tense and Release Exercise: Get in touch with your sexual energy with this powerful practice. Begin by sitting comfortably on the floor. Just as with the heart breath, begin by relaxing your jaw and opening the back of the throat. Allow the inhale and exhale to happen as naturally as possible without force while still allowing the greatest flow of air in and out of your lungs. Find a focal point in front of you and stay with your breath, letting the added oxygen charge your body. You may contract your PC muscle to begin moving erotic energy as you breathe, but stay with your breath for at least ten minutes. When you're ready for the release portion of this tense and release technique, take twenty to thirty fuller, faster breaths and lie back on the floor. Take three full breaths, holding the third. As you hold the breath tense every muscle in your body, especially your stomach, bottom and PC muscle, which is the one you'll be strengthening through Kegel exercises (see Section 5). I like to press into the floor. Tense and hold for fifteen seconds or longer, then release. Stay open and expanded, allowing energy to move. Enjoy!

Affirmation: I am open to the power within me.

Solar and Lunar Breathing

We here in the Western World tend to take breathing for granted unless there's a problem, such as allergies or asthma which hinders the process. The ancient yogis studied the science of breath (pranayama), understanding its vital importance and usage as a powerful tool. This formed the basis of Hatha Yoga. Hatha is comprised of two words "HA" (breath of the sun) and THA (breath of the moon). It was observed that breath sometimes occurred through one nostril and other times the other. It is believed that this is linked to celestial influence and where the moon is passing at a given time. Many Tantric texts claim that through balancing the solar and lunar breath, one can free themselves from the influence of destiny.

I have found solar lunar breathing to be incredibly helpful for concentration. It is both relaxing yet energizing. It can also reduce nausea and stress. It is said to purify the energy body after three months of daily practice with it. I highly recommend trying it for at least a week. It's a tool you'll be glad to have in the tool chest, so I've included it here for you.

Solar lunar breathing exercise: (also known as: alternate nostril breathing)—this takes some practice, if you've haven't done it before. Be patient, and it'll flow after a few attempts.

Sitting upright, spine straight. Get comfortable, and relax the mind. Close your right nostril with your right thumb or index finger by pressing on the right side of your nose. Inhale air through your left nostril. Hold the air for a few counts, but not for longer than is comfortable. Exhale through the right nostril. Close the left nostril with your left thumb or index finger. Inhale through the right nostril, holding the air for a few counts, but again not longer than is comfortable. Exhale through the left nostril. Continue alternating for a count of twenty retentions. Repeat morning, midday, afternoon and evening.

Affirmation: I find balance through my breath.

Section Three: Playing with Energy

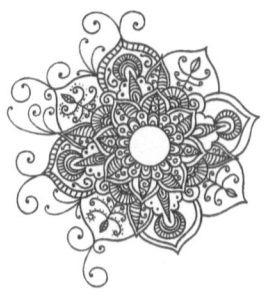

"Energy work is priceless. It makes every day extraordinary and transforms the mundane to the holy."
—Silvia Hartmann

Setting your Sexy Space

With our busy lives, it can be especially challenging to shift gears and slip into a sexy mood. Eastern philosophies encourage setting the mood by creating a welcoming, sensual environment. When the energy of the room is pleasing to the senses, it will be easier for you to feel comfortable in your explorations. I will refer to this erotically enhanced environment as your sensual space, but you may think of it in whatever terms are comfortable for you. It's time to get sexy. What does your fantasy space look and feel like?

Find what works for you. By setting this sensual space, you are investing in creating a pleasing environment where you feel comfortable and safe to experiment. Setting your space can be fun, and doesn't require a lot of time. It should add a sense of romantic warmth to the environment, through textures, colors and scents that are pleasing to you and your partner. Your space should be nurturing to you while also inviting exploration and passionate play.

Some simple ways to set sensual space are through the addition of fabrics, pillows, candles, incense and mood music. It is always nice to add draped sensual fabrics, but please make certain they are not near heat or fire. The additions of plants, flowers, and other organic materials are also recommended. You may want these to have a symbolic meaning for you, such as adding well-placed roses to infuse the energy with love, or orchids or irises to represent sensuality. Dimmed lights quickly lend a sensual mood, so perhaps you want to include a couple of low light lamps to the room. I always love to light candles to set the mood.

The ancient Indian texts even describe the type of bed one might use for optimal love making. A bed should be firm but soft, so one can move up and down delightfully, and be large enough so erotic activities can be uninhibited and free. Also recommended is a bed with columns and curtains, turning your bed into a small separated room that sets the mood and delights the senses. Similarly, you can hang drapes, silk or even a mosquito net around your bed to enhance sensuality. A well-equipped bedroom has small and large pillows. A half-moon shaped pillow can be used to support the buttocks of a woman. You may also want a small soft pillow on which she can rest her head. Find shapes, textures and sizes that work best for you and your beloved.

Exercise: Create a sensual space for yourself, or add special touches to the area where you'll be doing the practices in this book. What pleasing scents and luscious colors appeal to you and your beloved? How can you bring the sexy into the room in ways that inspire you to play and feel delicious?

Affirmation: My surroundings support my explorations and growth.

Energy and What Science Understands

There's nothing new under the sun. None of the concepts that I'm introducing are new. In fact, moving energy for healing and pleasure is one of the oldest practices in the world. There have existed healers since at least 4000 B.C.E. who have understood that our health is a direct reflection of the quality of the energy flowing through our bodies. Modern day science is catching up to these old philosophies and current scientific evidence supports Eastern philosophy's descriptions of these energies. In

Ancient India this vital life force energy is called "Prana". It is known in Chinese medicine as "Qi" or "Chi". Our personal energy field, which can and has been measured, extends beyond our physical body.

While we as human beings like to perceive things in a way that relates to our belief systems, there are concepts we've learned to take for granted, despite not fully understanding how these things work. For example, we cannot see electricity, we all know that it works, and appreciate its benefits. If you are not yet familiar with thinking of yourself as an intricate energetic system, that's perfectly okay. Most of us have become so familiar and comfortable with the Newtonian physics-based explanations of the world around us that a limited view of the structure of the material world has become second nature. It is easy to think of the things around us as dense matter. The table and chairs seem to be solid, right? But scientific experiments of the past few decades suggest that matter does not have any set basic building blocks, and that on the subatomic level all is mutable and interconnected. Quantum science has determined that at a subatomic level, everything is 99.99999999% empty space. In order to understand these subatomic particles, scientists measure it as units of energy. Everything, yourself included, is conscious energy in motion. Physicists tell us that the universe is comprised of a single unifying, interwoven energy.

Tantric texts have referred to the human energy field as the subtle body. The subtle body is a measurable energy field, which Eastern philosophies have described as a part of an interconnected web of transmutable energy within the universe at large. And, modern scientific research is confirming this perspective. It is important to have a basic understanding of your energy body in order to use the Tantric-based energy exercises that I describe throughout this book. I've found that the more I have become aware of myself as energy and learned to move this energy in my body, the more incredible my potential for pleasure has become. It was not my mind frame when I began using these practices, and I wish I had understood it more. If it feels like a stretch, just pretend, and continue on.

Scientific evidence is increasingly pointing to the reality of the universe as a non linear, expanding potential. Our world is always in motion, an expanse of dancing, and pulsing particles of light, energy, and information. In the early 19th century, physicists Michael Faraday and James Clark Maxwell investigated interactions between fields. Their electromagnetic field theories describe the universe as having fields that produce forces that interact with each other, and explain the subtle, vibrating light. Fields have been defined as a condition in space that has the potential of producing a force. Unlike the old Newtonian view of two particles attracting each other, for example, physicists found that a charge affects the space around it. You've probably experienced that your thoughts, words, and actions all make an imprint on the energy field around us, but there is plenty of scientific evidence for it too.

Let's look into the research a little more. The energy patterns around plants have been well documented, and illustrate the potentials for human energy fields, as well. While it's not well known or accepted in the United States, all biological systems generate coherent patterns of light called biophotons. Russian scientist Alexander

Gurwitsch developed detectors to sense such light in the 1920s. For the past three decades German scientist Fritz Popp has researched biophotons extensively. In his studies, he observed that parts of an injured plant carried greater levels of biophotons, seemingly in an effort to heal itself. Photons create a gigantic field, which unifies all of creation, as described by unified field theories. This human energy field, or subtle body, is described in similar terms in Eastern teachings.

There are various types of subtle energy fields. Human energy fields, like plant biophoton fields, are capable of exchanging energy and information. That empty space that's being measured as energy units is a holographic field that carries information for the growth, development and reproduction of the physical body. This is an extension of David Bohm's hologram concept, which holds that all pieces, no matter how small, are an exact representation of the whole. Researchers have learned that our energy field also communicates information that correlates closely with our health. There are hundreds of studies documenting bioelectromagnetic effects on molecules, cells, organs and beyond, yet few physicians or scientists, much less members of the public, are familiar with this research. It also reflects what we've known since childhood, as we witnessed that a cut, burn or other injury healed on its own. Our body has its own intelligence which is always working toward optimum health and wellness. We can support this through various practices, such as covering things with a band aid. But, there are other amazing tools available to us to support energetic imbalances which form through negative thinking and emotional baggage we carry through life.

An electrocardiogram, or EKG, can measure the electromagnetic fields of the heart. Similarly, an electroencephalogram, or EEG records the brain's electromagnetic field. There are also magnetic fields produced by electrical activities of the brain and heart that are measurable using what is termed as a SQUID (or, superconducting quantum interference device). The fields of energy produced by the brain and heart interact with every cell and molecule in the body. In the 1930s Harold Saxton Burr researched electrodynamic fields surrounding humans, trees, plants, and other forms. For forty years he detected and measured these fields, which he called "L-fields" (the "L" stands for "life"). Burr maintained that these electromagnetic fields are like a jelly mold for the form, and that an abnormality in the human field can provide warnings of things being out of balance within the body. Robert Becker, an orthopedic surgeon in New York has been researching electromagnetic fields and has established the relationship between regeneration and electrical currents in living things.

The ability to tune into our own energy field is a powerful skill. Of the energies with which we're comprised, sexual energy (called jing chi by Taoists) is the most potent, and can be consciously cultivated, moved around the body, to revitalize our lives. This also feels really amazing! This is one of the most important secrets of the Tantric tradition.

New research around heart resonance shows that the heart has an intelligence all its own, similar to the brain. The power of the heart shouldn't be underestimated. It is a powerful healer. When we consciously shift to an energetic mode that is heart centered, that energy comes from love and kindness, and can allow for powerful healing to take place first within our own energy field. That loving energy is also mirrored back by the universal energy of which we're all a part. Did I lose you there? I hope not, but I'll provide practices to help you experience these things later on. Just remember that the key is to be gentle and loving with yourself. Nothing is taboo in Tantra, so reserve judgments and enjoy the ride.

A basic concept in Tantra teaches that the human body is a mirror image of the universe. These philosophies state that each of us carries the patterns of the entire universe in our DNA. It is believed that our sexual experiences embody and grant us access to the mysteries of the cosmos. We are a microcosm reflective of the whole, containing both masculine and feminine energies, much like the positive and negative poles described in science. Tantra offers ways to integrate and come into balance with these energies, and therefore with the universe as a whole. It has been my experience that our body can also serve as a source of connectivity and transcendence.

While it may seem like a strange or new concept, people have known for thousands of years that coming into oneness with a partner allows an opening to the interconnected energy fields of the universe at large. The practices I detail will teach you to become more sensitive to these energy fields. The intensity of this process is best approached with gentleness, and self-love. It has been my experience, and much has been written confirming my experience, if we do not have self-love, that condition is carried in our energy field, and is mirrored back to us by the experiences and people we attract into our lives. For, how could we expect another to love us when we do not love and approve of our self first? You attract what you unconsciously think you deserve. When you use the exercises I detail in this book, approach them with an attitude of love and compassion for both yourself and others with whom you may be sharing them. While it may seem esoteric or cliché, love is the true essence of our being.

Exercise: You may or may not be consciously familiar with your energy field, but we're going to play with this a bit now. Bring the palms of your hands together and rub them back and forth quickly for thirty seconds. Feel the heat generated. Now slowly move the palms away from each other and feel the energy field between them. Keep moving the palms away from each other slowly and notice when you no longer feel that energy field between them. Now take your right hand, palm facing down, and place it a few inches above your left arm. Experiment by moving it closer and farther away from your arm, never actually touching skin to skin. Can you feel the energy field around your arm? How much distance does it extend? Continue to play with getting to know this field around your entire body each day.

Affirmation: I am connected with the energy of the Universe, the essence of love.

Being Present

Many philosophies, experts and books speak to the importance of being in the now, or present moment. With greater concentration you'll be able to see better what's really happening in any given moment. It's easy to get caught up in the melodramas of life, especially in our fast-paced society. I purposefully remind you throughout this book that by being in the now fully, you will be in your place of greatest power, in the flow with the universe, with access to your strongest intuition or guidance system. You won't have to second guess yourself about things. You'll just know.

The Knowing

There is a knowing, which cannot be explained,
Deep, visceral, quivering, at the core of your being
When you try to put your finger on it
The knowing eludes, escapes
Just outside the periphery
Of clear as day logic.

—Antonia Hall

When you live with your attention in the present moment, you will also become more aware of your energetic body, which is a constant barometer registering important emotional reactions in the body. Tantra and science explain this phenomenon as an energy exchange between your own energy and the energy of the people with whom you come into contact. Energy flows between people, which is why you may find yourself connecting well with some people and not others. Often times people choose to tune out these messages, instead allowing their thoughts to drift away from the situation or moment, or even holding their breath to numb out the emotional reaction they don't wish to experience. By staying present with these internal communications you gain a valuable source of information that will serve you well in many types of situations.

Let's further discuss the potent potentials of true presence. As you start using Tantric-based exercises you will become more sensitive to the subtlest sensations of the energy body, and you'll become adept at moving energy around the whole body using deep breathing and visualizations. Moving energy into specific parts of the body with intention is a powerful tool for awakening ecstatic potentials, healing body, mind and spirit, and is a necessary skill for living a multi-orgasmic life.

Our energy body, like the physical body, is an intricate system, always working to maintain balance and harmony. By bringing awareness away from mental chatter, and into your core, you can better preserve and regenerate your energy. Leaving too much energy in the mind is unhealthy, and leaves one depleted and potentially irritable. One of the best ways to shift this is through breathe. With conscious breathwork you'll learn to bring awareness into a particular body part, while infusing your body with new energy, and also opening to experiencing greater levels of pleasure leading to multi-orgasmic experiences and full body orgasms.

Exercise: Choose a place where you will not be interrupted, preferably in the sensual space you created for yourself. Sit or lie comfortably, spine straight. Relax your jaw and breathe normally. Watch your mind, without judgment. We tend to live in our minds, moving to the next thing on the 'to do' list, in the future, or in the past, or replaying an exchange we've had with another. Shift your awareness to your breathe in the present. Feel the air as it makes its way into your lungs. How does your chest and belly open to make room for the air? Keep breathing, experiencing the intricacies of the stages of inhalation and exhalation. Don't make yourself wrong when mind chatter tries to take over, taking you away from breathe awareness and the present moment. For so many of us monkey mind chatter has become habitual. Become aware of when you're allowing old mental tapes to run on autopilot. Observe the process with amusement. You are beginning a process whereby you are taking back control of your powerful life energy, rather than continuing to let the autopilot run things. As long as you stay with the willingness to return to the present moment and your breathe, you are succeeding. You may want to set a timer to ensure you've sat with breathe for at least ten minutes. Keep doing this daily over the next week, without judgment, experiencing the present moment anchored by your breath.

Affirmation: I stay in the present moment, mindful of the valuable information available to me.

How Energy Moves Throughout the Body

The medical community in the Eastern World views the circulation of life energy throughout the body as essential for health and well being. When there are stagnations or blocks in the energy field, there is disease. Once the natural flow of energy is restored, rejuvenation and renewal takes place, physically and mentally. As I discussed in detail in the last chapter, the human body has bioelectric energy in every cell in the body. This energy moves in circuits, known as meridians, throughout the energy body. If you've ever been to an acupuncturist you are probably familiar with these concepts, as acupuncture's focus is the regulation of energy through these channels.

Did you know that the body's circuitry is comprised of a back and front channel? When unhindered, energy flows up the back channel and down the front channel. The back channel begins at the perineum and runs up the spine to the crown of the head around the front of the forehead and ending at the indentation above the upper lip. The front channel runs from the tip of the tongue, down the throat, and along the middle of the front of the body back down to the pubis and perineum. Touching the tip of your tongue to the palate behind your top teeth acts as a way to close the circuit. Closing the circuitry allows you to move energy around your body through these channels in a circle throughout your body. When you are finished circulating energy around the body, you can store it in the abdomen (see diagram). This is a powerful and delicious multi-orgasmic skill to have.

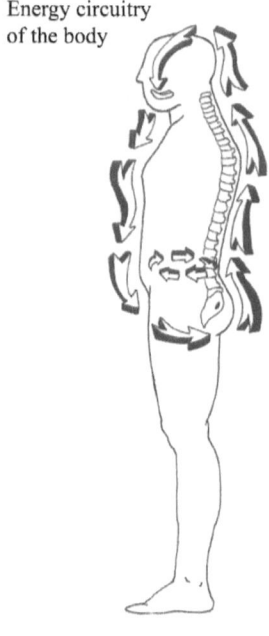

Energy circuitry of the body

When you consciously begin moving energy throughout your body it may feel like a tingling sensation, prickling, pulsing, or buzzing. This is all normal. If you're more practiced, you may experience a rushing sensation. Remember to keep breathing deeply and slowly during the practices. Never try to push or force energy to move. Energy moves with focus and intention. This may seem far out, but scientific studies such as biofeedback have confirmed that with focused attention, an increased activity can be seen in the nerves and muscles. Being able to bring awareness to your own energy body and the movement of energy through your circuitry is essential to becoming multi-orgasmic and successfully integrating the full-body orgasmic techniques. Trust me, it's very worthwhile.

You are surely familiar with the feeling of your own

sexual energy. When you become aroused and those sexually hungry feelings arise, you are cultivating your sexual energy. Now you are going to tap into the incredible power of this energy by drawing it up from your genitals and circulating it throughout your body. This is the basis of multiple and full-body orgasmic practices used by people for many thousands of years. Not only is it incredibly pleasurable, but you will also be energetically revitalizing your body. You will learn to gain control over your sexual energy, which is powerful for men and women. Men seem to appreciate the liberation gained when they find new control over their bodies, deciding when to ejaculate instead of feeling at the affect of their (often) untimely conclusion. Women love the freedom of having different types of orgasms, which flow in continuous waves, felt throughout the body. It's my experience, confirmed by others who utilize these techniques, that this energy carries over into your everyday life, sparking creativity and helping one stay healthy in body, mind and spirit.

You may experience an increase in sexual energy once you begin these practices. Remember to circulate your sexual energy throughout your body, to keep yourself in control and balanced. I recommend that you always begin each day with a grounding exercise. I'd also highly recommend grounding prior to any the practices I describe. It is also important to use the non sexual healthful practices, such as meditation, exercise, eating well and drinking plenty of water. All of these become increasingly important during this process. Take care of yourself to really reap the benefits of a multi-orgasmic life!

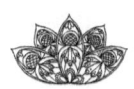

Exercise: Lie comfortably on your back, letting your breath become a natural flow, in through your nose, out through your mouth. Imagine your body's internal circuitry, visualizing how energy flows through it from the base of your spine, up the back channel to the top of your head, and down the front channel. Don't force anything. You're just bringing an awareness to it.

Affirmation: Energy flows effortlessly throughout my body, healing and revitalizing me.

What is Tantra and the Tao?

The more I have studied and practiced Tantra, the more respect I have for these sacred texts, and the information they impart. What a shame that it has gotten such a bad rap here in the Western World. Tantra emerged in Asian society as an uprising against a patriarchal regime that stressed sexual abstinence as the only way to reach enlightenment. Tantra is not a religion, but a philosophy that wanted to grant freedom from religious indoctrinations. As the earliest forms of Tantra were passed down directly from teachers to their students, the precise dating of the origins of the lineage is difficult to pinpoint. There is evidence that the origins of Tantra go back at least to the Indus Valley civilization, known today as the Harappan culture. Deriving from the root word *tan*, Tantra means "to weave, expand, extend or stretch" and has been interpreted to mean "to weave together" and "that which expands understands". The philosophies of Tantra were adapted into Hinduism and Buddhism, which spread when they were carried from India to neighboring areas, such as Tibet, Mongolia, China, Japan, Cambodia, and Indonesia. More recently, they have emerged in the Western world.

The original Tantric masters sought not to renounce and detach from the bondage of existence, but to step more deeply into it, transforming all acts into a connection with creation and spirituality. They posited that sexuality is a way to reach enlightenment, and that it was possible to do so in a single lifetime. Tantra provides a way to weave spirit and matter, enabling practitioners to achieve their fullest potentials in all areas of life.

Tantric practices offer ways to get in touch with sexual energy, and use it for healing, transformation and, ultimately, greatly improving one's well being. Tantra is a philosophy, a science, and an art, which has been practiced and carefully handed down for many thousands of years. It allows one to consciously use one's inherent sexual energy to enhance life. It has been my experience that through embracing and expanding into this energy, one's life can shift into a state of everyday ecstasy, or what I call a multi-orgasmic life. It is transformative, healing, powerful, and very pleasurable.

The sacredness of female form as sexual vessel of the divine is especially evidenced through Tantric art and texts. The dancing goddesses in ancient art works, revered as the source of life, are similar to images of women dancing ecstatically in cave art found in the Upper Paleolithic era. This is also evidenced by yoni lingam statues, art representing the sexual joining of male and female depicted through a phallus (lingam) inside a vagina (yoni). These statues have been found around the globe. I saw evidence of this during my visit in December 2011 to Pura Tirta Empul in Bali, Indonesia, a temple that dates back to 926 C.E., which has a large yoni lingam statue inside the main Holy Temple.

From the ancient Europeans of the Upper Paleolithic there is evidence of goddess worship, attunement with nature, affirmation of the female form as sexually powerful and sexuality as a gateway to divinity. We also see evidence of ecstatic rituals, such as dancing and sexual rites. These themes are echoed in Tantric texts and art. The use of rituals involving dancing and copulation can be seen in both the Paleolithic art and Tantric traditions. These bridge sexuality with spirituality and, I would posit, allow for a human experience of transcendence. One does not need to embrace this belief to enjoy the benefits of the techniques.

When the ancient Tantric practices traveled to China, they were assimilated into the Tao, a philosophy which later became a religion. The Tao (pronounced "Dow") translates to "The Way" or "Path", and offers ways to live, from medicine to sexuality to cooking. Most of the techniques I offer are Tantric based, and some are Taoist adaptations.

Tantric practices are not just a way to have huge full body orgasms and hours of great sex, the techniques offer a pathway to allow one's everyday life to become infused by ecstatic energy, and this arrives through practices that may surprise you. The Tantric texts detail a way of life concerning the foods we eat and drink, bathing, sleep, breath work, massage, meditation, yoga, and other various rituals. It has been my experience that the more of these practices you're willing to incorporate into your life, the greater the rewards of experiencing enhanced pleasure and life fulfillment. Throughout these Tantric techniques, sexuality is consistently brought to bear as it relates to everyday life. In the Eastern world, sexuality has been considered both an art and science to be studied, practiced and passed down as sacred teachings. When we embrace our inherently sexual nature as human beings, we can experience ecstatic states and transcendence, through which our lives are nourished and enriched.

Exercise: The word 'Tantra' alone can bring up feelings for people, especially in the Western World. What does it bring up for you? Did reading about the history of the texts change your feelings toward it?

Affirmation: I embrace the wisdom inherent within me.

Circulating Energy

Our life energies have a natural flow. When they are circulated, they rejuvenate the body and mind. The stagnation of our life force causes disease and diminished energy in our daily lives. But, you can consciously circulate the energy to lend vitality to diminished areas. Proper maintenance of our life force energy is what makes all of the difference between the young and old, and why some feel age more than others. Once you become more aware of your energy field, you'll be able to circulate energy not just for yourself, but for your partner, as well.

In the chapter on becoming multi-orgasmic you will learn to move sexual energy throughout your energy body. You can continue using this basic exercise for some time first, or if you haven't had much experience with energy work. Once you're more familiar and at ease with the practice, then you can move on to the more potent sexual energy circulation exercises.

Circulating Energy Exercise: While standing, feet shoulder width apart, spine straight, ground and center yourself. Close your eyes, and find a comfortable, gentle and rhythmic movement. You can step forward and back, or rock, or gently bounce from the knees. Keep the body moving harmoniously. Become aware of your center, at your navel. Feel your vital energy swirling there. Allow your breathe to find a rhythmic balance, noticing the inhalation and exhalation. Breathe deeply, inhaling through the nose, and exhaling through the mouth. Focus on the energy moving from your navel out toward your arms and legs, letting your life force energy vitalize and re-energize your body. Move the energy with your breath, and know that your body will receive this energy.

Affirmation: Connecting with my energy's natural flow rejuvenates me.

Circulating Energy for Another

As all is energy, it is possible to not only move one's own energy, but also to move energy for your partner. Moving energy for a partner can be a very sensual and pleasurable experience. This is a powerful practice that can be combined with other activities. As always, show respect by communicating with your partner and making certain they feel comfortable with this technique prior to using it on them. Energy exchanges should always be agreed upon in advance.

Exercise: Have your partner stretch out, lying flat on their back. Stand, sit or straddle your partner. Breathing from your abdomen, visualize the flow of energy moving throughout your partner. Sweep your hands over their body while seeing in your mind's eye the energy filling the passageways of your partner, noticing where flow may be blocked or deficient. Hold the intention of relaxing and rejuvenating every area of their body. Ideally you will learn to become so comfortable with this practice, it becomes natural to exchange energy with each other during love making. When you become more accustomed to distinguishing between the subtle variations in energies in your own body, you'll be able to send sexual energy into your partner. Once you're more accustomed to the practice, moving energy for your partner can be done while touching them, engaging in oral sex, or while using a toy on your partner.

Affirmation: Exchanging energy is a beautiful expression of love.

Section Four: Physical Pursuits

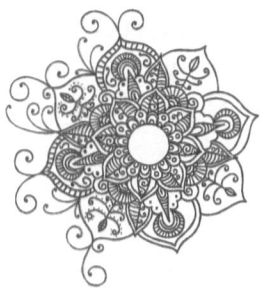

"I am convinced that life in a physical body is meant to be an ecstatic experience."

—Shakti Gawain

Anatomy

Sadly, many of us have never been taught the basics of how our bodies work, especially in regard to the body's sexual responses. We're expected to know how to please our partners, but every body is different. Sexual responses vary by individual. Explore by yourself, so you can go back and teach your partner what you learned. Adventure together, and be surprised by where the delicious journey takes you. Set aside all judgments, as always, for this sensitive play. We're going back to sex ed basics, because understanding your own body and your partner's body is sexy, and results in far greater pleasure giving and receiving. Isn't it unbelievable that we didn't learn this a long time ago?

Female Anatomy (The Yoni)

Every woman is different, especially where nerve endings are concerned, thus women get turned on in different ways. I've had friends confide that they're afraid to look "down there". But why would you let your partner be the only one to look at your intimate parts? Get to know your yoni, which is where your most powerful energy resides. Honor this, and enjoy it. Your sexual pleasure and orgasms are created in your body, the one you'll have for the rest of your life. It is imperative that you get to know what turns you on and gets you off. The female body is nourished and replenished through orgasm. Autoeroticism increases the flow of female (yin) energy. This is a gift and valuable resource. Let's get acquainted with the intimate anatomy of your pleasure center, so you can access its potential.

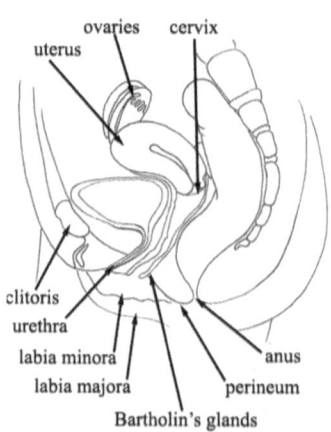

If you look in a mirror, you'll be able to look at your vulva and vagina. I'm sure you're familiar with the two larger outer lips (labia majora), which is usually covered in hair. The soft flesh inside these is the inner lips (labia minora), which is smaller, usually more sensitive, and soft, smooth and hairless. The color, shape, and sizes vary dramatically from woman to woman. We are each a unique flower. Isn't that lovely? The clitoral hood, a small flap of skin, usually hides the clitoral head. That's often the hub of the pleasure center because the tip of the clitoris has the most nerve endings, 8,000 nerve fibers, which is twice as many as the penis. The clitoris is the only organ in the body designed solely for the purpose of pleasure. Some women enjoy having the clitoris licked, sucked or played with, while others find it painful or overwhelming. The Tantric viewpoint believes that the clitoris is directly related to all of the glands in the body and stimulation improves hormone balance. All the better reason to play with it.

Recent research on the clitoris has revealed that it is far larger than once believed. This potent pleasure center was shrouded in mystery and wasn't examined internally until MRI's were done in the late 1990's, and sonography lent further understanding in 2009. That's a long held secret! What they discovered is that only about a quarter of the clitoris glans resides outside the body. This tip is much like the head of the penis, and like its male counterpart, also swells with blood and gets harder upon arousal. The internal clitoris consists of two wishbone shaped 'legs' called the corpora cavernosa, which can extend up to 9 centimeters in length. Just with all vaginas, the clitoris varies from woman to woman. About three in four women need clitoral stimulation to orgasm from intercourse. Stimulation is likely happening in greater ways than formerly thought. What's important is to know what feels most pleasurable to you, ladies.

The urethral opening is very small and often difficult to locate, but if you spread your inner lips you should see a small dimple between your clitoral hood and vagina. This important little pathway is where urine exits from the body. It also has nerve endings, which can be pleasurable or painful to have stimulated during sexual activity and lovemaking. Care should be taken when stimulating the urethral opening, as it can be easy to push bacteria into it which will result in bladder infections. None of us want those.

The vagina opening may be concealed by the lips. There is a ring of muscle just inside the vagina that is part of the larger pubococcygeus (PC) muscle, which we will be exploring in more detail in the next chapter. Just beyond this is the G-spot, first referred to by Dr. Ernst Grafenberg, which can be felt along the front wall of the vagina (belly side) a couple of inches inside. It is not always easy to find, but it is ridged tissue, and it swells with stimulation. Not all women may be able to find the G-spot, but they may find a similar intense pleasure spot in other places within their vagina, especially deeper inside. Explore and play, finding your personal pleasure spots.

Have you wondered about female ejaculation? Perhaps you ejaculate a small or large amount of fluid, also known as "squirting" or "gushing". Tantric texts refer to this fluid as "madhu", meaning honey, or nectar. This fluid comes from the paraurethral ducts, surrounding the G-spot, and is a combination of fluids from the Bartholin's glands, mucus from the top of the cervix and vaginal secretions. Blood vessels in the urethral channel fill with blood during sexual excitement, which can lead to the feeling of needing to urinate. While panic about this is understandable, it is very unlikely one would urinate while sexually aroused. If you want to learn to ejaculate, try having your partner stimulate your G-spot with firm pressure. The likelihood of success increases if you're already stimulated, so there's already ample swelling. When you feel that need to pee, push downward rather than tensing inward and upward, which tends to be a common inclination. Focus on your own pleasure over a specific outcome. If you're not immediately successful, keep practicing.

Another pleasure spot is located on the front of vagina wall (belly side) close to the cervix, and was noted by Malaysian sexologist Dr. Chua Chee Ann. While it takes long fingers, or a longer dildo or vibrator to find it, this ducts area can be reached and stimulated pretty easily during sex. In Tantric philosophy, all of the vulva and vagina are capable of bringing great pleasure and stimulating your energy throughout the body. In later chapters I will provide exercises to help move your sexual energy throughout your body. The body is capable of deriving orgasmic pleasure from all of its many parts. Do not be attached to having specific "spots", just enjoy the ones you have for now. The techniques in this book can allow for new levels of responsiveness allowing for new pleasure spots to emerge.

The fleshy dome at the top of the vagina is the cervix. A tiny dimple in the top is where fluids travel out, and sperm may enter. Amazingly, the cervix is made to stretch from the size of the tip of a ballpoint pen to encompass an entire baby passing through it. Some women may experience intense pleasure and waves of electric like sensations moving up their spine from having the area around their cervix stimulated. The cervix opens to the uterus, a hollow muscle which lies in the lower abdomen. The uterine walls contract and expand during intense orgasms, and can expand to nearly 100 times their original size during pregnancy. Isn't the body amazing?

The ovaries are two small glands found on each side of the lower abdomen. The ovaries produce eggs during the menstrual cycle and also produce female hormones. They are considered to be a powerful resource for women in Tantric philosophy. Breathing exercises using the ovaries as a focal point is said to nourish the woman's energy source and reduce aging.

The perineum is the skin between your vagina and anus. There is a network of blood vessels and part of the PC muscle beneath this skin, which swell during sexual arousal. The anus contains the second highest concentration of nerve endings. Anal stimulation and penetration can be very pleasurable for some women. Because the anus does not secrete its own lubrication, like the vagina does, it is very important to use plenty of lubrication for anal play. I recommend buying a lubricant made specifically for this purpose (see the chapter on lubricants for more information). Both male and female bodies fill with blood from front to back, so anal play is more likely to be pleasurable if you're already well stimulated. Begin with fingers or smaller toys until you are used to anal play. It takes some time. Never put anything that has been in the anus into the vagina or other body part without washing it first, or bacteria exchanges will likely lead to infection.

Male Anatomy (The Lingam)

Every man has a unique size, shape, and color lingam. Your sensations and what feels best to you also varies. Unless you're already having multiple and full-body orgasms, you've yet to tap into your greatest sexual potential. Let's get acquainted with the intimate anatomy of your pleasure center further, gentlemen.

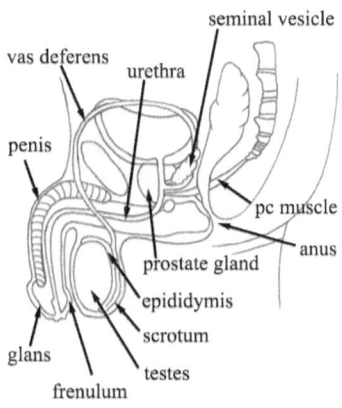

The penis, testicles (testes) and prostate gland comprise most of the male genitalia. The penis is made of spongy tissue, and contains no bones or muscles. The penis extends for two to three inches inside the body in the pubococcygeus (PC) muscle, which can be strengthened in order to achieve stronger erections and orgasms, and to obtain better ejaculatory control (explained in detail in the next chapter). There is a small tube that runs through the center of the penis called the urethra, which carries urine and semen out of the body. When a man is nearing readiness to ejaculate semen, a valve shuts off the pathway to urine. The head of the penis, called the glans, is very sensitive due to many nerve endings. In an uncircumcised penis the foreskin covers the glans when the penis is relaxed, and pulls back to expose the glans when the penis is erect. There has been very little research and conflicting assessments about the number of nerve endings found in the foreskin and how circumcision may change sensitivity of the glans.

Just below the corona, or ring of tissue at the tip of the penis lies the frenulum. The frenulum is often likened to the clitoris, and is often very sensitive. Some men may have a small bump to indicate the frenulum, while others do not. Ask your partner to show you where this highly sensitive and often arousing place is located on his penis, and how to best stimulate it.

The two testicles (testes) are enclosed in skin called the scrotum. It is in the testes that sperm and male hormones are produced. A small tube, called the vas deferens, extends from each of the testes to the prostate gland. At ejaculation the semen is pushed through the urethra and out of the tip of the penis by contractions coming from the urethra and muscles in the shaft and base of the penis. The testes swell during sexual arousal and pull up tightly against the body. Pulling the testicles away from the body is one method of prolonging ejaculation.

The prostate, which is a chestnut shaped gland at the center of the pelvis behind the pubic bone and just above the perineum, is often quite sensitive. It is similar to the G-spot in women. Both male and female bodies fill with blood from front to back, so it takes longer for the prostate to become an arousal point. This often occurs as the man approaches orgasm. It is important that a man is well aroused prior to prostate play, which can be done (carefully) through the perineum, anus, or both simultaneously. Ejaculation from the prostate is usually flowing rather than in spurts, and may produce more ejaculate. Like the G-spot versus clitoral orgasm in women, the prostate orgasm can be more intense and may result in a more emotional sensation than just a physical one. Men can also experience simultaneous prostate and penile orgasms, which may result in a full body orgasm.

Due to the high concentration of nerve endings in the anus, and its close proximity to the prostate gland, it can be a very pleasurable area to have stimulated for men. Enjoying the stimulation given through anal touch is normal, natural, and does not in any way indicate that you are "dirty" or have homosexual tendencies. Being gay is an orientation, not a practice. Having different sexual orientations is a normal part of nature, in humans and other species. As long as you are honest with yourself about your natural predilections, there is room for it in Tantra, where anything goes as long as it's done with mutual respect.

Exercise: Go into your sensual space, or other place where you will not be disturbed. Turn off phone ringers, or other potential distractions. Get out a mirror and really explore your intimate parts. Admire the colors, textures and shapes that comprise your yoni or lingam. Get to know your intimate parts more intimately.

Affirmation: I love and embrace the doors to my sexuality.

Getting to Know Your Body More Intimately

In addition to knowing your mental, emotional, and spiritual sides at a deeper level, it is important to know your physical body as well. The physical form is the vessel that carries us through life, yet most of us have never taken the time to really get to know our bodies intimately. Treating your physical form with respect and appreciation is another important concept in Tantric teachings. The Tantric viewpoint sees the physical body as a microcosm of the universe. Out of respect for the divine, the body is to be kept clean and healthy. In my opinion, treating yourself with the compassionate loving care with which you deserve to be treated just makes sense.

Through daily rituals of self-care, you can connect with yourself at a deeper level, bringing about increased feelings of self-esteem and well-being. When we are in a new relationship, we go out of our way to make that person happy. I am suggesting that you begin a love affair with yourself in this same way. Start to add new self-care treatments to your day, bring awareness to the activities revolving around your body's care, and take time to explore ways to give your body more pleasure.

These physical practices also require that you become more present and aware in the moment. We can oftentimes go into autopilot throughout the day. Instead of absent-mindedly showering off, become aware of the warm water as it gently caresses your body, feeling your muscles relax. Consciously touch yourself with loving care. Smooth a layer of delicious organic coconut oil all over your body, admiring your unique shape. Gods and Goddesses come in all shapes and sizes. Life is too short to go around carrying societal judgments around with us about our physical form. Ideally, the body reflects the loving care we have offered it, and if your body doesn't feel and appear well-loved it may be good to ask yourself why.

Exercise: Be brave in your explorations. The best way to cultivate awareness of your sexual energy is through self-pleasuring. Do you find that you have judgments around this activity? Most of us have been taught to think of self-pleasuring as dirty, shameful or a bad thing that, at the very least, shouldn't be discussed. Add to that the common societal belief system that pleasure is shameful unless received by one's partner, and we find ourselves in a powerless structure completely at odds with our inherent need for pleasure and desire. It is time to rethink this important self care-giving practice.

Tantric philosophy sees self-pleasuring as a genital exercise and a source of knowledge. Through self-pleasuring a man can learn the rhythm of his sexual arousal, using techniques to practice non-ejaculation, and moving sexual energy throughout his body for full body orgasms and better health. Women can self-pleasure to revitalize their bodies. Many of us have trained ourselves to masturbate quickly, focused upon an end goal. Take your time, cultivating pleasure and knowledge of your body. Both men and women can learn with conscious awareness what turns them on, so they can explain these desires to their partner. Pay attention to touch, pressure, locations, and what feels best. Notice the feel of your potent sexual energy as it rises. Understanding your cycles of your arousal is an essential practice toward becoming multi-orgasmic.

Affirmation: I love my sexuality and it loves me back in magnificent ways.

Fit is Sexy (and Feels Great)

The body is made for movement. The body wants to move. And, the more you honor its need for movement, the better you'll feel, physically and emotionally. If you already have a regular exercise routine that works well for you, that's great. If you don't, it probably bothers you. We all know we feel better when there's a proper exercise routine implemented into our lives. There are lots of types of exercise to choose from, and it's time to find a form that works for you.

Physical exercise is a great way to get in touch with the body. Not only does it make you feel great (endorphins), it'll decrease your stress levels, and increase blood flow. This is especially helpful in adding heat to your bedroom activities. In fact, if you want to be able to utilize the techniques you've been learning to the fullest, you'll want to have a regular exercise routine. Tantra has some incredible positions that will allow you and your partner to experience incredible mind bending pleasure for great lengths of time. Sadly, these will be far more challenging if you're out of shape. Think of what a hot, sexy couple you'll be!

It's important to balance physical activities that offer your body aerobic training and flexibility. Yoga provides a way to lengthen and strengthen your body, and also prepares the body for Tantric lovemaking practices. As one might expect, research confirms that physical exercise not only has many health benefits, but it also aids lovemaking.

Exercise: If you do not have a regular exercise practice, I want to encourage you to begin one. Balance it with your yoga practice. Don't have a yoga practice yet? Really?? Okay, on to the next chapter then, please.

Affirmation: Being fit feels fabulous and sexy.

Why Yoga Matters

The teachings of yoga have readily made their way to the West, and it is vastly understood that yoga has health benefits for both the physical body and mental well being of the practitioner. Yoga means to "join together" or "make union". Yoga allows one to join together their individual consciousness with the infinite consciousness of the Universe. I remember telling my Western doctor that I'd begun to do yoga, and he said that was great exercise for me. I stopped, looked at him and said, "It's so much more than exercise." Yoga allows us to come into balance with our masculine and feminine energies, transcending duality and accessing the infinite mind of which we're all a part.

Yoga provides postures called "asanas" (meaning a position that is firm and pleasant), through which one can stretch and tone the physical body and soothe the nervous system. It is also a wonderful practice to reduce stress and rejuvenate your body, and a tool through which we can promote health and well-being. It is not recommended that one practice yoga when sick, or after heavy meals or exercise. Also, women should not practice inverted postures while menstruating. The best times for yoga are early morning and early evening. Between ten minutes to half an hour per day is a sufficient practice. Do not over do it. More is not necessarily better. Take it easy. If you're a beginner, know that it takes some time to develop a yoga practice. You will not, and should not expect yourself to turn into a pretzel from the start. Never push the body, and don't let others, even a teacher, tell you to do something which you know is too much for yourself, or could cause injury.

There are many postures, and some will come more easily than others for you, if you're new to the practice. Don't get discouraged. Many of the yoga asanas are named after flowers and animals from which they were inspired. Yoga is a potent practice through which the practitioner can come into balance and access his/her higher self. It's an important tool for excelling at your lofty goal of living a multi-orgasmic life.

If you're reading this and thinking, "But I can't even touch my toes. How can I do yoga?" Let me first remind you that you can touch your toes, you just need to bend your knees. Hamstrings only stretch so far, and touching your toes in yoga is about lengthening the spine. Every beginning has to start somewhere. Keep things simple, letting go of attachment about where you are, and appreciate the benefits, which are brought forth really quickly. I've started over from the beginning many times with my yoga practice, and am always surprised by how quickly my body is willing to allow for renewed flexibility.

Yoga is more than stretching and breathing, it is a conscious discussion between yourself and your body. Investing in a positive relationship with your body is worthwhile. Stay open, receptive, and let your body speak to you. Enjoy the slow gentle stretching. Connect with your breath, and let it guide you toward getting to know the subtle energies in and around your body. Visualize the flow of energy in each posture. The body is resilient and wants to be open and expansive. Many of the yoga asanas were developed to allow healthy flow of these energies. You'll feel great, and be present in your body. I'd be surprised if even a small amount of yoga each morning didn't increase your energy levels noticeably enough to turn you into a believer pretty quickly.

Yoga will prepare your body for ecstatic experiences and the intricate Tantric positions you'll want to explore at some point. A well stretched, limbered body really contributes to a great sex life and can also help prevent potential injuries.

Exercise: If you do not currently have a yoga practice, I'd like you to begin. Try some simple asanas to begin, such as sitting poses, cat posture, or even corpse pose, on your back. You'll be amazed how quickly you'll begin to flow from one asana to the next. Also, yoga will energize you, so you can do more each day. If you're already a seasoned yogi, renew your love and appreciation for yoga by trying new asanas, and devoting yourself to an ever expanding regimen.

Affirmation: I stay flexible as I go about my day.

Nourishment

The physical body is an intelligent and amazing system, but it can only do so much with the fuel put into it. We all know that eating fruits, vegetables, and whole grains is better for us than eating processed or fatty foods. Yet, it can be easy to take the body and our current health states for granted without considering how our sustenance (or lack thereof) is effecting us internally. As you embark upon living your best, most multi-orgasmic life possible, I recommend exploring which foods provide you with the most energy and make you feel good. Did you know that many people are actually allergic to dairy and wheat? Many of my friends have discovered that a few dietary changes decreased or eliminated health issues they'd had. The Yogic texts counsel eating in moderation and at the same scheduled times each day, which many Western doctors agree is best for proper digestion. I have found that eating foods that are in season is the most sustainable and healthy way to provide the body with healthy sustenance.

Experiment with eating more fresh, locally grown fruits and vegetables to get the nutrients your body is intrinsically craving. It is best for your body, the environment, your local farmers, and the planet at large. Buy organic whenever possible to ensure that you are not adding additional toxins into your body. Our environments are often polluted with poisons found in the beauty products, cleaning supplies, and foods we consume. By purchasing certified organic foods and products you can rest assured that they were not grown with pesticides or herbicides, and that they are not genetically modified or irradiated. Limit your intake of toxins by buying organic and in season, and you'll be providing your body with better nourishment.

It is equally important to drink plenty of fresh, filtered water. Breath and energy work can help you clear energy blocks you may have carried for years. Providing your body with the proper nutrients and lots of extra water cannot be overstated. There are no easy answers as to how much water each person needs on a daily basis, but it's been my experience that extra water is necessary when practicing these techniques. Let your body be your guide, but remain conscious of the requirement, which will probably exceed what you're used to.

Tantra also notes the uses of food as an erotic experience. Sharing in a sensual light meal and glass of wine with your lover prior to lovemaking can be a delicious way to connect. Taoists recommend eating until satisfied but not too full. It is inadvisable to engage in sexual activity after a heavy meal. Tantric texts also advise avoidance of strong foods such as onion, garlic, peppers, and also fatty fried foods, heavy meats, and eggs.

Exercise: If you haven't been to your local Farmer's Market, look it up and attend the next one that fits into your schedule. If one is not available, find the next best source of local organic produce. If this is already a way of life for you, then purchase some fruits and vegetables you've never tried before. Make a special meal for yourself with awareness that food is the supporter of life, and that you are caring for your body in the best ways possible in your commitment to living a multi-orgasmic life.

Affirmation: My body thrives when I provide it with healthy nourishment.

Stillness and Nature

I have mentioned the importance of bringing awareness to the interconnectivity of all of life. Each part exists as a smaller part of the larger whole, which is also a core teaching in Tantra. One of the most enriching ways one can experience this connectivity is by getting out into nature. Surely you have noticed that a journey to the mountains, beach, or other favorite nature spot recharges and energizes you. We are uplifted by nature. We're rejuvenated and healed.

Rush. Rush. Rush. More people are living in urban communities now than ever before. In a society of doers and achievers, we can sometimes forget the importance of slowing down. The body needs stillness, and when combined with soothing natural surroundings, we are nurtured physically, mentally, and spiritually. Dance with nature for a day or week, and you will return to daily activities a more rested, nurtured version of yourself. Every once in awhile it is very important to get away into nature, unplug and enjoy. There are many types of nature adventures from which to choose, any of which is apt to decrease stress and revive your body and spirit. Journey to the beach, lake, river, mountains, desert, or whichever form of nature is calling to you.

A fast way to build energy reserves is to meditate outdoors. The natural world around us has vital energy that you can tap into, even if you are a city dweller with limited natural surroundings. So add time in nature to your daily 'to do' list. Even if you can only go outside, stretch your arms to the sky and drink in some sunshine or fresh air for a few minutes. Even short daily visits with nature will rebalance and serve your well-being.

Exercise: Go out and explore a local nature spot. Have you always meant to visit a neighboring mountain trail or lake? Spend as much time as your schedule will allow out in nature today. Notice how it makes you feel.

Affirmation: I am at my best when I take regular Nature breaks.

Types of Touch and Sweet Spots

Whether or not it leads to sex, the art of touch and massage are an appreciated gift to give your partner, especially if they've had a rough day. Set the mood in your sensual space or set the mood in a warm room where you won't be disturbed. Warm your massage oil (almond oil, jojoba oil, apricot kernal oil or coconut oil work well) between your palms, then approach you partner gently, keeping your strokes fluid. Your hands should move over their body effortlessly, otherwise replenish your oil. Ask your partner to guide you in what feels good, and if there are particular areas they'd like for your to work on. Tantric philosophy says that the more in tune you become, the more pleasure you'll derive by giving pleasure to your partner. This has been my experience, and those of other Tantrics' I know. Play with giving and receiving pleasure, and you may find that you can orgasm simply from witnessing your partner doing so.

Basic Massage Strokes:

These basic techniques can be easily mastered, just practice until you find a blending that works best for you and your massage recipient. Be careful to work on each side of the spine, but never on the spine directly.

Circles – Your circles can be smaller, or larger. Move your palms away from the spine, using your palms or fingertips, trying to keep your movements balanced on both sides, so that your hands mirror each other in a synchronized fashion.

Effleurage – These long gliding strokes are done with the palms, fists or forearms. This is a very soothing stroke, which warms and relaxes the muscles, and relaxes the mind, body and nervous system.

Kneading – Lightly squeeze then release fleshy areas with curved palms. This is a great way to release tension. Be mindful that you aren't pinching the skin.

Petrissage – Using the pads of your fingers, apply a gentle circular motion to release tension. This is particularly helpful along the spine, where knots can form.

Tapotement – With the fingertips or soft fists quickly drum, tap, or hack (using sides of hands) keeping a rhythmic tempo. This technique helps to stimulate the nervous system, circulatory system and musculoskeletal system, stimulating weak muscles and loosening tight ones.

There are certain sweet spots which shouldn't be ignored. The head and shoulders are a great place to begin or end your massage. The head has lots of nerves, and a head massage alone (using the pads of your fingertips) can be a great de-stressor that feels great and will leave your partner smiling. Tracing down the length of the spine using light pressure that increases can be incredibly sensual and pleasurable. The neck is a sweet spot for many of us, and can be massaged to release tension or licked and nibbled to increase arousal.

The hands and feet connect with every other part of the body, and should be carefully stretched and massaged. Working between toes and fingers can be very sensual. Bend the knees and work up the calves from the ankles, then you may wish to move between the thighs in rhythmic movements to excite your partner. The groin and inner thighs are a sweet spot for many men and women, but can also become ticklish, so be conscious of the amount of pressure you use. Perhaps your partner prefers a flicking tongue or little kisses trailed up their thighs.

The nipples are a sweet spot for many men, as well as for women. Tease around the nipples first, circling inward in smaller spirals until you reach the nipples. Roll the nipples gently, teasing them between thumb and forefinger. Lick around the nipples, teasing the hardened nipple with the tip or flat of your tongue. Every man and woman is different, so get to know which breast and nipple are more sensitive and what pressure brings the most pleasure to your partner.

Moving down the belly is a delicious way to raise arousal in your partner, teasing along the bones of the pelvis before moving toward the sex organs. Fixating on genitals as an exclusion of the rest of the body is never recommended. The giving of pleasure through stimulation of the genitals is an individual process, as sensitivities vary. Brushing your lips against, flicking and swirling your tongue over, and suckling on genital regions, beginning further outward and moving inward is usually most pleasing. Using fingers at the base of the penis while sucking it, and to tease inside the vagina while licking the clitoris can bring added pleasure for many.

Guys- if your partner is a woman, try thrusting your fingers along the front wall of her vagina a few inches inside to stimulate the G-spot. You may be able to feel the little ridges there. Gently hooking fingers and pulling back a little (this is subtle) while thrusting against the front wall can bring powerful orgasmic pleasure. Be careful while learning this technique, and make certain you have clean hands and short nails before putting fingers inside your sweetheart.

Exercise: Take turns massaging each other, even if it gets spread out on different evenings. Be sure it's scheduled, so you both can anticipate when one will be giving and when one will be receiving. Ask your partner what felt good, and what things they could have done without. Learn how to touch and please each other in new ways.

Affirmation: My love flourishes when I exchange conscious touch with my partner.

Sensory Experiences

The journey to a multi-orgasmic life is one whereby partners make a commitment to bringing more pleasure into their lives and that of their partner. It is awakening to the sensual side with which we were all born, and a dedication to appreciating the deliciousness that can be found in the seemingly mundane, or what has become routine. Connecting with your senses is a huge part of this. When eating, experience your food, the smell, taste, textures and love with which it was created. When touching your partner, use more than your hands to give pleasure, including feathers, your hair, soft silky materials, velvet, leather, or cool glass, ice cubes, a heating pad to heighten senses and increase arousal. Speak sweetly to your beloved, whispering words of appreciation and devotion to their beauty.

Exercise: In this sexy exercise you will rely upon your sense of smell, touch and taste, which may be amplified once your visuals are subdued by a blindfold. Take at least thirty minutes per person for this exercise.

For the person stimulating your partner's senses, gather all of the sense play items beforehand. Perhaps you'll want to blindfold your partner just outside the sensual space, then lead them in. Make certain your partner feels warm or cool enough, and is sitting comfortably. Lean in and whisper in their ear about the erotic journey through the senses you'll now be taking them on. Tease your partner's sense of sound for about ten-fifteen seconds, with an equal amount of time kept in silence between each sound. This helps build anticipation, and thus excitement. Move on to sense of touch, tickling and teasing the skin of their neck, arm, legs, hands, and face. Move slowly, keeping a similar time frame for each new object, and the anticipatory time between. Lastly engage your partner's sense of smell and taste. Be gentle, kind, playful and respectful of your partner, who has willingly submitted for both your pleasure.

Affirmation: My body is wired for many types of pleasure.

Toys and Lubricants

There is plenty of evidence that sex toys have existed for thousands of years. The dildos of ancestors past have taken lots of creative forms over the years and we now have many options today. Toys offer additional pleasure-giving experiences for men and women, solo or partnered. Bringing toys into partnered play should be viewed as a welcome way to expand horizons, rather than a replacement of connectivity or a sexual issue. Toys can bring new excitement, and can lead to more connectivity and pleasure for both parties. If you are not using toys with your partner, approach the topic honestly, with compassion, a sense of wonder, and excitement at the joys they can bring forth for you both. Communication is best, with an assurance that there will be respect for boundaries. This can be an exciting way to spice things up, and there are lots of different types of toys out there to explore.

Some Types of Sex Toys:

Dildos are an artificial penis. Dildos can be used alone, or with a strap-on. Dildos come in a multitude of shapes, sizes and materials.

Vibrators come in various shapes, sizes, and speeds. Some are shaped like a penis, an animal, a wand, or a hand. They may vibrate (as the name indicates), rotate, and thrust. Butterfly is a type of vibrator, shaped like a butterfly, the main portion of which lies against the clitoris to stimulate her. They can be worn under clothes, and some come with a remote control. Eggs can be inserted into the vagina or anus. These egg-shaped, or bullet-shaped vibrators come with a remote control. The finger massager are another type of small (silicone) vibrator held with a finger against the clitoris, anus, or other body parts to send shivers through you or your partner. They commonly come in varying speeds. The couple's vibrator is worn during intercourse and stimulates her G-spot while enhancing pleasure for him as he moves in and out of his partner.

Benwa balls are traditionally made out of metal, but can also be made out of other materials, including plastic, silicon and semi-precious stones. These balls are placed inside the vagina. Movement causes them to clink together. The vibration against the vaginal walls stimulates delicate nerves.

Penis rings (aka cock rings) are placed around the base of the penis and behind the testicles during an erection to trap blood flow, increasing the erection and sensitivity. There are different styles of cock rings, beginning with a single strap, ones that separate the testicles, and vibrating rings (couples' rings) that stimulate the clitoris during intercourse. Cock rings shouldn't be worn for more than twenty minutes at a time.

Butt plugs are usually made from hard plastic or silicone. Butt plugs are usually smaller dildos, which are used to stimulate the anus in men and women, and the prostate in men. Anal vibrators and anal beads can also be used for this purpose.

Make certain to play safely with your toys. Never use a toy anally and then insert it vaginally or orally. Be sure that your toy is clean and has no rips, tears or imperfections that could cause injury to delicate tissues. Use a lubricant (discussed below), and condoms or dental dams on your toys if they are being shared. Always express to your partner if something doesn't feel good, hurts, or pushes you beyond your comfort levels.

Cleaning your toys properly is essential for the prevention of bacterial infections and diseases. Many types of sex toys can be washed with a soapy washcloth using an antibacterial soap that's gentle and won't cause irritation. Or, sex toy cleaners can be sprayed on and wiped off. The cleansing process depends upon what your toy is made out of, and all toys are not created equal. My advice is to invest in high quality toys, and avoid any cheap rubber and plastic toys that contain phthalates, which have been shown to be harmful to health. If your toy has a fruity fragrance or sweet smell to it, it's probably contains phthalates and is not worthy to be placed in your body. If you're unsure, err on the side of caution and wrap that toy up in a condom prior to use. Always unplug toys prior to cleaning them.

How to Clean Your Sex Toys:

Toys made from glass can be washed with soap and water. Avoid high temperatures.

Stainless steel toys can be boiled or placed in a 50:50 bleach-water solution for ten minutes. Many stainless steel toys are also dishwasher safe.

Hard plastic shouldn't be boiled. Soap and water is the best cleaning option.

Silicon dildos can be boiled for five to ten minutes. Silicon toys can also be placed in the top rack of a dishwasher or cleaned with soap and water.

Silicon vibrators shouldn't be boiled as you can injure them. Wash them with soap and water.

Nylon toys can be washed with a gentle anti-bacterial soap.

Cyberskin and vinyl toys are porous and care should be taken when washing them. Use warm water and allow them to air dry. A small amount of cornstarch can be applied to keep your toy from getting sticky.

Leather should be cleaned with leather cleaner, or a damp soapy cloth. A layer of leather conditioner can be applied to keep your toys at their best. Never soak leather. Apply a thin layer of clear nail polish to metal parts to prevent tarnishing.

Lubricants

All bodies are different, and we all go through various cycles in life, due to hormones fluctuations, diet, stress, and other various reasons. It's normal and natural for some women to need more lubrication. There is no reason to irritate your delicate parts with rubbing, friction, or worse, pulling from trying to insert things. There are various types of lubricants readily available at many stores to assist with adding sweet moisture to your play. But, it's important to know what ingredients they contain so you don't harm yourself or break down condoms, sex toys, or your diaphragm.

Ladies! The vagina has its own intelligence, and continually works to keep itself fresh, healthy, and balanced. Women can nurture and support this process by allowing it to breathe by avoiding tight synthetic clothing, harsh soaps, and perfumed products, including laundry detergent and dryer sheets. Douching and other deodorant products will mess with your pH balance, causing new problems, and are best avoided. Some women are also allergic to Nonoxynol-9 and other spermicides. If you have continued pelvic pain it is best to see a doctor.

Making things slick with lubricants feels great for both men and women. There are three types of lubricants: water-soluble, silicone-based, and oil-based lubricants. I prefer water-soluble lubricants without glycerin (which can cause irritation for some women), as it is most like natural lubrication, can be used safely with sex toys, and can be easily washed off. Water-soluble lubricants don't stay wet as long as silicone-based lubricants, but they're the the least likely lube to cause irritation or infections, and you can always add a little saliva to refresh them.

Silicon-based lubricants have to be washed off with soaps or cleansers. Some people find silicone-based lubricants to be irritating. Oil-based lubricants (such as oil, vaseline, lotions, or Crisco) are not advised ever, as they can cause infections and will break down latex, making them a dangerous combination with latex birth control such as condoms, diaphragms or cervical caps. There is also evidence that they can cause an imbalance for women's delicate system, much like vaginal deodorant products. Flavored lubes can be fun, but can also cause yeast infections due to their sugar content, as can any sweet additions to the bedroom. Sugar on top rather than in is probably going to be better for your delicate parts.

Exercise: Explore new lubes for bedroom play. There are many different types of lubricant, and variety can be fun. Many companies make similar formulas in different varieties. Purchase one you've never tried before.

Affirmation: I delight in exploring new ways to please myself and my partner.

Rhythms

Just as there is a rhythm and flow to life, there is a rhythm and flow to successfully thrusting inside your partner. While pornography likes to portray men quickly and forcefully thrusting into their partner, this technique will lead to fast ejaculation and is unlikely to leave your beloved sexually fulfilled. Be sure that your partner is ready, as it usually takes some time for a woman's vagina to lubricate, swell and for the cervix to move back to make room for your penis. Tantra describes patterns of blending shallow and deep thrusts to enhance pleasure for you both and increasing likelihood of successfully prolonging ejaculation. I know this is yet another thing for you to learn, gentlemen, and that you probably don't want to have to count during sex, but I assure you that these techniques work really well, and just as with the breathing and energy practices, this will all become second nature. For this you will get your Sexual Superhero cape, dear sir.

When you alternate between shallow and deep thrusts, be careful not to pull out of your woman completely. The deep thrust pushes the air out of the vagina, which creates a vacuum. The shallow thrusts intensify the sensations within her, which she will love! The balance between the two types of thrusting will lead to more orgasms for her, and will help you prolong. Find a rhythm, so that you don't have to focus too hard or become rote in your technique due to counting. Alternate between nine shallow and one deep thrust. Once you become more adept at prolonging ejaculation, you can reduce the shallow thrusts to six or even three (with greater mastery). Nine is the yang (masculine) number, considered to be magical.

Another nine count thrusting technique, which I would find challenging to count out personally, involves alternating your thrusts for different counts each time. The key to this is adjusting counts. So again, find a rhythm that works for you, enhances pleasure for you and your partner, and assists you with prolonging undesired ejaculation. This thrusting technique begins with nine shallow, one deep thrust. Then eight shallow, two deep, seven shallow, three deep, six shallow, four deep, five shallow, five deep, four shallow, six deep, three shallow, seven deep, two shallow, eight deep, and one shallow, nine deep. My best wishes to you. They work, I promise.

There are nine types of movements a man can make while thrusting into his lover. First is Moving Forward, whereby the lingam is moved forward directly into the yoni. Second is Churning, with the lingam in hand, it is turned and churned inside the yoni. Thirdly, one can use Piercing, with the yoni lowered and the upper yoni is struck by the lingam. In Rubbing movement the lower part of the yoni is pierced with the lingam. In Giving a Blow, the lingam is pulled mostly out of the yoni then forcibly thrust into the yoni. Blow of a Boar movement involves a rubbing of one part of the yoni with the lingam. When the lingam is moved up and down while deeply inside the yoni without being removed, it is called the Sporting of a Sparrow. Pressing the lingam deep inside the yoni is called Pressing. Lastly when the man and woman alternate pushing the lingam and yoni together without removal, it is called Pressing Together, and can create a quicker climax.

Exercise: Experiment with various rhythms. If you're coupled, discuss how different rhythms feel to you both. If you're single, play with a toy that represents your favored partner's genitals, experimenting with various rhythms. What feels best to you? Does your favored rhythm change as you become more aroused?

Affirmation: I invite greater rhythm into my multi-orgasmic life.

Soft-On Sex

It is a fallacy that men must have an erection to make love to his partner. Sometimes a woman doesn't want a hard penis inside of her, but a soft shaft and energy exchange can provide great pleasure and stimulate orgasms. I've had plenty of orgasms from a soft penis inside of me. This can be highly erotic, tender and beautiful.

Soft-on sex: Making certain that she is moist and ready, get on top of your lover or lie side by side. Create a circle at the base of your penis using your thumb and forefinger. Gently squeeze. Slide your penis inside of your partner and gently thrust, keeping the ring with your fingers at the base of the penis. Contract your buttocks and PC muscle, focusing on moving the sexual energy throughout your genitals, into your lover. Your lover may want to arouse you by kissing you, nibbling your ears, and playing with your perineum, testicles or anus. Some erotic talk can be great here, as well. You do not have to thrust and force love making for this to be a highly erotic and pleasurable experience. You may both just want to lie very still, penis inside the vagina, and breathe together. Perhaps you'd like to amplify things by moving energy throughout your energy body. This can create even more passion between couples than you might imagine.

Affirmation: My partner and I can connect deeply without expectations.

Positions for Success

While it isn't necessary, you may want to invest in a copy of the Kama Sutra so you can explore the many positions described there. Some positions will require a mastery of yoga and acrobatic abilities. Release the need for completing them all, and enjoy playing with the possibilities. When a woman is on top, it is easier for a man to control his ejaculation, so you may want to utilize this position more as you learn the practices that will lead to your becoming multi-orgasmic. This position can also allow women to stimulate her G-spot, and find her own rhythm.

While man on top, known as the missionary position, may seem boring and unimaginative, it allows for connectivity between partners, who can eye gaze, kiss, and use breathing exercises together easily from this position. Adding a pillow beneath the woman's buttocks will aid in shifting penal stimulation to the highly orgasmic potential deep within her, to the side of her cervix. Just be careful not to hit the cervix, which can cause pain and cramping. Try alternating shallow and deep thrusts, and when she is fully aroused and (hopefully) experiencing orgasms, you can shift her feet up on your shoulders for even greater pleasure. This can lead to mind-bending multiple and full-body orgasms. Try using a breathing technique so that you are sipping the air in and out as you might through a straw, ladies. Wow!

After a more rigorous and energetic time of love making, a couple may want to lie side by side to cool off and connect. This position doesn't allow for deep penetration, but does allow for G-spot stimulation and sweet intimacy. Be careful not to be thrust out as she climaxes. Once those PC muscles of hers become strong, there is a greater tendency for this to occur. Continue to breathe consciously, and perhaps you'd like to move energy together.

Having the man approach the woman from behind can be highly pleasurable for both parties. I recommend placing a pillow under the chest of the woman and having her rest forward on it so she is angled. This allows for good G-spot stimulation and can lead to lots of multi-orgasmic pleasure for both of you. It is difficult not to have eye contact, but looking over your shoulder at your man occasionally can be even more erotic and sexy for you both.

Many prefer the Yab Yum position, which is a sitting position. The man is in a sitting position, similar to lotus pose, and the woman straddles him. It is recommended that lovers wait at least a half an hour into love making to get into this position so that energy is open and flowing. This position can be energetically intense, but allows for deep intimacy. The woman can move up and down on her lover, but this position also allows for beloveds to simply be still and move energy together. The woman squeezes her PC with in and out breath. Some people have described feelings of transcendence, seeing colored lights and a sense of leaving ones body in the Yab Yum position. You may experience tremors, shuddering and Kundalini energy rising up the spine. Release expectations and just enjoy the deep feeling of love and pleasure that can arise here. Move slowly, shifting positions slightly, as there are many amazing variations that can be found from here.

Exercise: Choose a sexual position you and your partner have never tried before. Experimentation in the bedroom (and other places) keeps things fresh and fun. Keep practicing!

Affirmations: I enjoy exploring new ways to bring increased pleasure into my life.

Section Five: Orgasm Wisdom

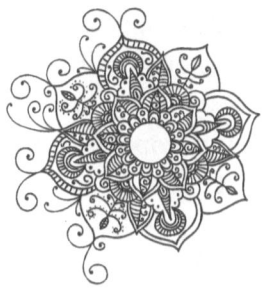

"An orgasm a day keeps the doctor away."

—Mae West

The PC Muscle

Many of you may already be familiar with the pubococcygeus (PC) muscle. Both men and women have a muscle that runs from the front at the pubic bone ("pubo") to the tailbone or coccyx. The PC muscle, also referred to as the sex muscle, is essential to your becoming multi-orgasmic, and is the muscle that you will be strengthening daily from now on, if you're not already. Trust me. A strong PC can make you very multi-orgasmic and a happy man or woman. Squeeze, release, strengthen, every day. Let's look at how this can be done for both men and women.

The PC Muscle for Women

You may already be familiar with, and even doing Kegel exercises. Kegels involve strengthening the pubococcygeus (PC) muscle, which next to the brain, is the most essential muscle to sexual pleasure. If you are unfamiliar with this pelvic muscle group surrounding your urethra, vagina, anus and pelvic organs, locate it by stopping your flow of urine the next time you are urinating. Squeeze this muscle to start and stop the stream of urine a couple of times and get a feel for its location so that you can begin contracting it on a daily basis.

Strengthening this muscle is easy through Kegel exercises, named for Dr. Arnold Kegel, a gynecologist who developed the exercise for women who were experiencing incontinence after they'd given birth. Kegel exercises require little time investment to be effective, and can be done anywhere. A stronger PC muscle will lead to better orgasms, as well as the ability to extend orgasms and move sexual energy throughout the body in enjoyable ways. Additionally, when you become more familiar and comfortable with this sex muscle, your partner will appreciate the way it squeezes him when he's inside of you during lovemaking. Contracting your PC muscle improves blood flow to your pelvis, generates sexual energy, and adds to natural lubrication. In the chapter on sexual positions, I also detail some positions through which this muscle can be maximized.

Squeeze to Please Exercise: Begin lying down or sitting at the edge of a chair. Insert two fingers inside your vagina. Squeeze your PC muscles around your fingers then relax. Spread your fingers, keeping them relaxed but at a distance from each other. Take a breath, exhale and relax. Now contract your PC muscle again and see if you can bring your fingers together, holding the contraction for a count of ten. If not, don't worry, as it just takes practice. Repeat two more times with a ten count hold.

It takes about two months to tone up the PC and begin noticing improvement in your sex life from its toning. More reps will shorten this time period considerably. It has been my experience that strengthening this sexual muscle will allow a woman to reach orgasm with muscle control alone, which is well worth the daily effort to achieve.

Kegels – Begin by contracting your PC muscle, inhaling as it tightens, hold the breath then relax as you exhale. Ideally you will be able to do twenty reps per day, with a ten second hold with each rep. Add reps as you get comfortable with the practices, but don't try to add too many at once. As with any new exercise, ease into this one, as it can be a painful area to have overworked.

PC Pump – When you are more comfortable with the basic PC exercise, you can progress to a PC pump. As with the basic PC exercise, you will tighten the muscle with the in-breathe, hold it for six-eight seconds, then bear down as you exhale. Practice for a few minutes each day. This is another hugely beneficial exercise for lovemaking, and great for women who would like to learn to ejaculate.

PC Pullups – Take a breath and relax your PC muscle. As you exhale, contract your PC muscle, pulling it upward. Repeat 9-18 times. Then contract your PC muscle for ten seconds while breathing naturally. Repeat three times.

The PC Muscle for Men

Like women, you too have a pubococcygeus (PC) muscle that runs from your public bone to the coccyx. Also like women, this is an essential muscle to exercise in order to become multi-orgasmic. When strengthened you will have stronger erections, more intense orgasms, and have better ejaculatory control. If the penis is not used regularly it can actually withdraw into the body. Sex organs, just like regular muscles, need exercise. The PC muscle is the sex muscle, and between learning your arousal states and strengthening your PC muscle, you'll learn how to orgasm without ejaculating and be multi-orgasmic.

The PC muscle, which surrounds the prostate gland, is like a valve around the genitals. Orgasm builds from the prostate, so learning to develop these muscles is imperative to becoming multi-orgasmic. It also has the added benefit of preventing prostate issues, such as hardening and swelling. One in seven men will get prostate cancer in their lifetime. It's important to do all you can to keep it healthy, if becoming a sexual superhero wasn't enough motivation for you.

If you are not familiar with your PC muscle, you can become aware of it when you push the last few drops of urine out next time you urinate. If you have a strong PC muscle, you should be able to start and stop the flow of urine midstream. Unfortunately stopping the flow of urine midstream may cause a stinging sensation initially. This is normal, and will remedy itself within a couple of weeks. If it continues after a few weeks, then you may have an infection and it is best to see your doctor for treatment before continuing.

Your PC exercise is similar to the women's but will be done while you are urinating. Inhale and contract the PC muscle to stop the flow of urine. Exhale and start urinating again. Repeat three to six times or until you no longer need to urinate. To add an extra intensity to this exercise (recommended, but not necessary), stand on your toes or balls of your feet and keep your teeth clenched during the exercise. Standing on your toes is like adding a little weight to the exercise, and clenching your teeth helps increase saliva, which cools the system and will help you gain control over ejaculation (as guided in later exercises). Remember that your efforts will benefit yourself and your partner both in truly awesome ways.

PC Pullups – Take a breath and focus on your PC area. As you exhale, contract your PC muscle, around your prostate and anus. Inhale and relax, releasing the PC. Repeat 9-36 times. Begin with lower reps, and work your way up, as this is also a muscle that is uncomfortable to have overworked for men.

PC Weights – You can add some resistance to your PC exercise once the muscle has been adequately strengthened. Ideally you will be able to raise and lower a towel on your erect penis. Begin with a washcloth and work your way up. There are also weight sets available for sale, should that appeal to you.

Exercise: It's important for these exercises to become a part of your daily routine. They don't take much time to carry out, and can easily be incorporated into your day. I cannot stress the importance of PC workouts enough. Trust me on this one. You'll thank me later.

Affirmation: I delight in becoming more attuned with my inner strength and power.

Orgasms

Men and women orgasm differently, so I've separated this section.

Orgasms for Her

Orgasms feel different to every woman, and feel different at different times for the same woman. Every woman orgasms differently, almost like her own orgasmic fingerprint. Sometimes orgasms arrive in a soft gentle wave, and sometimes they are like rocket ships sent off into space. They often differ for the same woman at different times, especially dependent upon how they're derived. Like men, there is a rising desire, increasing physical arousal, and orgasmic release (resolution). Orgasm is the peak experience that follows arousal. During arousal genitals fill with blood until the contraction of the PC muscle and vaginal walls brings pleasurable sensations to the woman. Women have an almost limitless potential for orgasm, and their bodies are wired to be nourished by orgasmic pleasure.

The vast majority of women who have never experienced an orgasm can learn to do so. At first, experiment with bringing yourself pleasure, and try not to put your focus on orgasms. Touch yourself, and introduce a toy or two into your experimentations. If you can bring yourself to pleasure through touch or playing with toys, you can learn to orgasm during sex. You may need to stimulate your clitoris while your man is inside of you in order to experience orgasm during sex, especially at the beginning of learning these techniques. But the more you practice breathwork, moving sexual energy throughout your body, and the other techniques I describe, the easier it could become to find orgasmic pleasure.

I have more good news for you, ladies! Research shows that our expectations largely influence our potentials for orgasmic pleasure. Moving through limiting mindsets that may have played a part in the lack of ability to reach sexual release will help you a great deal, as our beliefs greatly influence outcomes. If we expect to be able to orgasm for many ongoing minutes, we are more likely to have that occur. What are your goals? To come in succession- one orgasm after the next? Or would you prefer to have a long continuous orgasm? I recommend them all, but full body orgasms are my favorite. Also, the more types of orgasms you learn to have, the more you'll be able to shift into having the ones appropriate for a given situation. Perhaps you're enjoying a quickie with your partner, and just want one big O. Allow for it. All of this is possible, and the more you practice, the easier it'll become. Are you doing your breathing exercises each day? Are you exploring and learning what pleases you? Studies show that multi-orgasmic women choose techniques that they've learned work for them. Additionally, they're then better able to communicate these needs to their partner. Combined with your intentions, breathing exercises, and learning to move your sexual energy around, the body will all assist with these possibilities and soon you can be a Multi-Orgasmic Goddess.

Orgasms for Him

You may already experience multiple orgasms, but studies show that many men are not even aware of their body's multi-orgasmic potential. Especially in the Western World, many men are focused upon "getting off" and don't believe there could possibly be a better way to climax than the way they've been doing it for years. But, this is a limited perspective in which the fallacy that orgasm and ejaculation are the same thing. They're not. And, once you begin learning how to distinguish between these two processes, you'll be able to begin learning the secrets to becoming a Sexual Superman capable of orgasming without ejaculating, thus continuing to have intercourse with your partner, while bringing that pleasure into your body to experience big full-body orgasms. Imagine being able to extend that (average) six second orgasm, stretch it out for minutes, experience it throughout your entire body, and keep going, only to orgasm again and again. You will find new levels of sexual ecstasy you didn't know was possible, and probably become one of (if not the best) lover most women have ever had. Though with great (sexual) power comes great (respectful) responsibility, gentlemen. Always be kind, honest and respectful with your partner. Let's discuss some of the fun facts of your orgasmic potential, and later why ejaculating as you probably have been could be draining and potentially harming you.

Back in the 1940's sex researcher Alfred Kinsey discovered that over half of all preadolescent boys were able to have more than one orgasm without ejaculating, and nearly a third could have four to five orgasms in a row without ejaculating. This multi-orgasmic potential seems to get lost to the satisfaction found in orgasm in adolescence, as most men do not know that they have this ability in adulthood. Newer research has realized that orgasm has more to do with a mental process than a physical one, in men and women, both. For both men and women orgasm is a peak experience. But, ejaculation is a reflex, an involuntary muscle spasm that is separate from orgasm. By using the techniques I detail next, you'll learn to distinguish between these two processes and be on your way to becoming multi-orgasmic. This is going to expand your repertoire in such amazing ways, and you'll experience even greater sexual satisfaction than you knew was possible.

While men can decrease the likelihood of getting

prostate cancer by one-third when they ejaculate five times per week, the Taoist and Tantric philosophy maintain that ejaculation drains a man of his vital life force energy. It has been shown that being able to choose to use non-ejaculation techniques has many health benefits. Men I know who use these techniques confirm that they not only have the ability to experience far greater pleasure, but they no longer ejaculate sooner than they'd like, so they can continue to please their partner, as well. Additionally, many men say they have far more energy than when they were ejaculating every time they were aroused.

Semen is a vital essence, and regulating this emission is considered a cure to disease and increased longevity. When a man forces ejaculation (common in the Western World, especially with quickie porn habits) he not only decreases his vital essence and energy levels, he can experience ringing in the ears, tiredness of the eyes, dry throat, and a sense of being worn out. The Eastern view sees this Western method of racing to climax and the physical collapse afterwards as harmful and unnecessary. But, the practices I detail here which have been handed down for many thousands of years, allow for sexual retention, continuing as one desires, and having full body orgasms. Just stay open to this and the Sexual Superman status; it's worth it, fellas.

Your decision to ejaculate or not is up to you. I am not saying that there is necessarily anything wrong with the way you're doing things now. I am just handing over keys for you to experience a very amazing upgrade. You will certainly benefit from learning how to control physical orgasms. And, it isn't advised never to ejaculate. In fact, exchanging fluids with your (monogamous, safe) partner has many health benefits. It is a balancing act, and finding what makes you feel best. Perhaps you want to ejaculate every few days, but still experience the orgasms on a daily basis. This will depend upon your age, health level, and personal preference. Remember that the main difference here is that instead of one intense (average six second) moment of pleasure, you'll be able to extend this for longer periods of time and the orgasms can be experienced throughout your entire body through full-body orgasms, instead of localized. You'll also be able to keep pleasing your partner, who is also learning to have incredible full-body orgasms.

Exercise: In a safe, uninterrupted space (preferable your sensual space), take time to pleasure yourself. Really take your time and try to touch and play with yourself in ways you never have before. Notice the energy rising as you get toward climax. What does that sexual energy feel like prior to and at the point of orgasm.

Affirmation: My orgasms are a fulfilling source of nourishment and pleasure.

Benefits of Sex and Orgasms

A satisfying sex life with a partner not only provides a wealth of physical health benefits, it offers many emotional rewards as well. Being in a committed relationship often brings increased feelings of security, which is amplified through intimacy. Making love with a partner leads to greater connectivity and sense of emotional well being. It also fosters enhanced trust, self esteem, and contentment.

When a couple is in love and getting along, they're more likely to have sex, and this leads to a beneficial cycle of happiness, well being, and increased commitment. Through engaging in a regular sex life together, people experience a greater sense of overall satisfaction and have an easier time relating with one another outside the bedroom. Desire for one another grows, and this enhances connectivity and leads to better flow in all areas of the partnership.

You already know that orgasms feel good, and can put a smile on your face, but there are a lot of health benefits from orgasm, as well. Sex is a fountain of youth activity. Orgasms reduce stress, elevate mood, and make you look and feel younger, healthier and happier. That's because regular sexual activity increases blood flow, resulting in lower blood pressure. Not only will you burn calories, you'll increase flexibility, muscle tone, and physical strength, especially as you move into the more advanced Tantric levels and positions. A regular sex life greatly benefits the heart, reducing chances of heart attack, especially in men. Orgasms lead to faster cell regeneration, helping the body heal faster on the inside and look better on the outside.

Couples who share in pleasurable play together are more likely to stay together. After sex, the body kicks out hormones that encourage partners to relax with each other. Sharing in the sweet, after-sex glow with your significant other allows your love to blossom further. Oxytocin, corticosteroids and endorphins are released by the body which leads to reduced pain, elevated mood, and a stronger immune system. The chemical oxytocin produces feelings of being in love, so people in turn feel more connected with their partners. These feelings of being more bonded with our partner, promote touch and affectionate behavior. This is amplified by dopamine production, which leads to feelings of trust and loyalty.

The body also pumps out lots of other hormones during sex. The natural histamines the body pumps out can relieve allergies, asthma and even a stuffy nose. Prolactin production amplifies sense of taste, touch and smell. Our DHEA levels peak when we are 25 years of age. Low levels of DHEA can lead to chronic disease, weight gain and bone loss. But during orgasms we experience a surge of DHEA, which also protects the immune system, may lower cholesterol, and promotes healthier skin.

Women experience an increase in estrogen, which reduces risk of breast cancer and strengthens the pelvic wall for better bladder control and a better sex life. When the pelvic floor is stronger, a woman has fewer cramps, and has an easier time birthing babies. Sex also gives her skin a beautiful healthy glow!

The more couples have sex together, the happier, more confident they are, solo and together. Coupled sex does wonders for each individual's sense of self. Numerous studies have shown that partners who have a positive sex life have higher self esteem and experience greater confidence in the everyday world. Further research studies indicate that a regular sex life supports mental health, which lends to a more cohesive, supportive, and healthy relationship. Connecting with a partner in a loving and tender way is a remarkable healer. The heart and old wounds can be mended through the gift of a healthy sex life in a deep, caring, and committed relationship.

Exercise: Take out your journal and list all of the ways that orgasms and great sex have helped you physically and emotionally. If you haven't been having a healthy sexual relationship with your partner, reflect back to when you were. How did that affect your relationship? How did this ripple over into your everyday life? If you don't feel you've ever truly experienced a meaningful and healthy relationship, make notes about what you feel has gotten in the way and what needs to be released for you to make the space to allow the deeply loving relationship you deserve into your life.

Affirmation: Sharing our multi-orgasmic potential together strengthens the relationship with my partner.

Full-Body Orgasms

Tantric sex focuses not on the genital orgasm, like most of Western culture, but on an orgasm that is brought into the entire body with breath, the PC muscle and energy work. It is far easier to achieve full body orgasms than one might think. With some focus, intent and practice, you to will be able to extend your orgasmic potentials into mind-bending amazing full-body orgasms. Like "normal" orgasms, or having a succession of orgasms (multiple-orgasms), full-body orgasms are experienced throughout the entire body. Full-body orgasms can vary from gentle waves to strong tremors and out of body ecstasy. It's been my experience that the more you learn to open yourself to the sensations and cultivate the practices, the more you'll be able to have control over the types of orgasms you have.

For both men and women, you'll need to become aware of your sexual energy, of how to circulate it throughout your body, and the role the breath plays. Then you'll be able to relax into the pleasure of feeling your sexual energy building. When orgasm is close, you'll learn to be still and allow for it. We learn to tense to experience pleasure, but is through surrender and relaxing that we experience pleasure with greater intensity. Tantra is slower than regular sex, with the addition of purposeful mindfulness. Let the pleasure move through you, using your PC muscle to raise and move the energy, and utilizing your breath to expand into it. Your body will vibrate, shake, and energy will rise up your core. You will experience incredible pleasure throughout the body, and especially up your spine. This is full-body orgasm. It is orgasm magnified intensely. It holds great potential not just for sexual satisfaction, but also for healing, energizing, and stirring creativity. One can expect it to spill over into everyday life outside the bedroom, stirring feelings of joy and sparking new creativity.

Gentlemen, instead of your six-second genital-focused orgasm, you will be able to delay ejaculation and have a succession of full-body orgasms instead. You'll experience amplified pleasure, without sudden sleepiness, and you'll be able to continue to please your partner, all without reciting a favorite lineup in your head in attempts to delay gratification. This new skill doesn't mean that you have to continue having sex for hours. If you had a long day at work, or life's responsibilities limit your time for intercourse, you can ejaculate as you always have, but it'll be when you desire. The power is now in you to decide how, when, or if you want to ejaculate. We're just adding a really awesome new skill to the toolbox.

Exercise: Discuss full-body orgasms with your partner. What does each of you think of this concept? Is it new to you, or something you've wanted to try for some time now? How does each of you feel it may change your current sex life? What are your hopes? Take turns talking about it openly. If you're single, make notes on what attracted you to the idea of learning to be multi-orgasmic, and how what you've learned thus far has had a positive effect on you.

Affirmation: Learning new skills empowers my life.

Becoming Multi-Orgasmic (For Men)

It will take you anywhere from a couple of weeks to six months to learn and master these techniques. Some men will need longer than others to master these practices, but once you've learned the techniques, they will become second nature. This is a short term investment into being multi-orgasmic for life. The greatest secret to multi-orgasmic lovemaking is awareness and stabilization of breath, thought and semen. You will be able to gain control of all three of these, allowing lovemaking and energy circulation to continue almost indefinitely. This in turn leads to transcendental ecstasy far exceeding any pleasure you've known. Are you ready to become a Sexual Superman?

First begin to recognize the phases of your erection. It begins with firmness, when the penis begins to become erect. Then swelling occurs, when the penis is firming but not yet hard. In the third stage the penis is hard and erect. In the fourth stage, the penis is very stiff and heated, and the testicles draw into your body. It is in the third stage that you'll best be able to control your ejaculation. You're going to become so conscious of your arousal stages, that you can learn when to pull back and recirculate your sexual energy, and when to relax and let go.

Breathwork for Retention: Keeping control over your breath and heart rate is an important practice in learning to retain ejaculation, and experience multiple and full-body orgasms. Learn this breathing technique while not aroused, then start utilizing in the play of learning retention. Remember that breath is a big key for both men and women. Multi-orgasmic lovemaking is best accomplished when the breath is deep, rhythmic and is drawn through the nose.

Sitting comfortably, relax your shoulders and let your hands rest on your thighs. Take a few breaths. Bring the palms of your hands to your lower abdomen. Inhale deeply through the nose. Experience the retention of breath and the way your belly has pushed outward. Exhale through the nose, feeling your belly move back toward your spine. Notice that your penis and testicles pull up slightly. Continue to breath deeply in and out in this manner for a 9 count- 9, 18, or 36 times. Relax.

Extra bonus tip: If you are aroused and are having trouble cooling your sexual energy, you may want to try visualizing breathing between your eyebrows. Breathing deeply (through the nostrils) with focus on the forehead helps to focus the energy up toward your brain, where you want energy to move and can help prevent ejaculation.

The Pressure Point: There is a pressure point, known as the Million Dollar Point, which can delay ejaculation and even prevent semen from spilling should you pass that point of no return. This technique for retention is called Classic of the Immortal. Pressing on this point while contracting your PC muscle and inhaling deeply at the same time is one of the oldest techniques.

The Million Dollar Point is located just in front of your anus. It may take some time to feel out the point, but you should be able to feel an indentation when you press on it. You'll be using your three middle fingers of your dominant hand. When you press up you should be able to feel your urethral tube, which expands when you near ejaculation. You want to push on the urethral tube with your middle finger and press on each side of the urethral tube with the other two fingers. Contract your PC muscle. This may decrease your erection a little, but if you've hit the right spot you will stop ejaculation from occurring. Breathe deeply, and try pulling the sexual energy away from the genitals and toward your brain.

It's important to massage the area later, contracting your PC a couple of times and circulating your energy back around in your body.

Scrotal Pulling: As I mentioned earlier, your testicles pull up toward your body just before ejaculation occurs. Using your thumb and forefinger, make a circle at the base of your penis, above the testicles and pull down firmly to prevent ejaculation.

Moving energy: While there are various techniques recommended by Tantric texts, the best way to prevent ejaculation is to move your sexual energy away from the genitals and up the spine. This can also allow you to have incredible full-body orgasms. You can do this while you are aroused, or move your sexual energy while you are not aroused. Remember that sexual energy is also the creative energy that can fuel your everyday life without genital stimulation. Just as for women, this is another powerful practice to enhance your life. You can move sexual energy up your spine, revitalizing yourself, body, mind, and energetically, and experience pleasure at the same time. Wow, isn't the body amazing?

Eventually, you'll be able to learn to do this and master moving sexual energy up your spine without being heated or sexually aroused. Touch your testicles with one hand until you feel that zing of sexual energy. Inhale and gently contract the PC muscle and imagine sipping the energy slowly upward. Exhale, relax, but stay with the rising energy mentally. Continue inhaling, tightening and exhaling and relaxing while sipping your sexual energy up your spine. You may need to rock your pelvis back and forth letting your chin bob up and down to help move the energy. Continue for five to ten minutes until you feel the tingling at the base of your skull. Touch the tip of your tongue to the roof of your mouth behind your front teeth to allow the energy to move throughout your body and back down into your belly where it is stored (as in moving energy throughout the body exercise). If you can't bring the energy all the way up your spine, just store it in your belly and keep practicing. Most men find this to be a pretty easy and effective exercise. Play with it daily and record your experiences in your journal.

In order to fully understand your pleasure cycles, the Tantric texts recommend self-pleasuring. Knowing your own body and what turns you on is important for both men and women. Self-pleasuring is not meant to take the place of partnered sex, it is meant to enhance it. This is an important part of learning your arousal stages and how to retain ejaculation. In Tantra one becomes more deeply aware of the sensations in one's body, so please set aside pornography for these exercises. This is an important part of mastering the retention techniques and learning to bring more pleasure and vitality into your body through multiple and full-body orgasms.

Exercise: Set sensual space for yourself, and make certain to remove any potential distractions or potential interruptions. Lubricate your penis and begin stimulating the entire penis. Don't just focus on the head, but the entire shaft as well. Lightly touch your balls, even if this is not a usual part of your routine. Take your time, this is not a race. You want to become more aware of the stages of your arousal and ejaculation. In the first phase the prostate contracts. These contractions are experienced as a pleasurable sensation or fluttering, which last for a few seconds. This is when the semen moves into the urethra. You may have a few drops of clear liquid drip out of the tip of your penis. You'll want to prevent the next stage in which the semen is released through the penis.

Explore your perineum and Million Dollar Point. Can you feel the indentation with your fingers? You're going to continue to bring arousal, but prolong ejaculation for at least fifteen to twenty minutes. If you're used to ejaculating in minutes, this may be challenging, but it's the critical point of being able to master these techniques. Once you can exceed twenty minutes, you've learned a new level of control. Stay with the explorations, bringing yourself close, then use the breathing exercises, PC or pressure point to prevent ejaculation and bring the energy back up your spine. Press the tip of your tongue behind your teeth, breathe through your nose deeply and become still. Stabilize your breath, holding it if possible, but without forcing anything. Keep your spine straight, tighten your PC muscle. If necessary press the index and middle finger of the left hand one inch over your right breast, which short circuits energy. Exhale and gnash your teeth together to produce more saliva, which cools and nurtures your body. If you experience orgasm without ejaculating, congratulations. This is the beginning of full-body orgasmic potential. If not, don't be disappointed, as these skills take time and practice. You are training yourself for your Sexual Superman status, so congratulations are in order regardless. Keep training, and you'll be finding new rewards every day.

Affirmation: I love that my body is multi-orgasmic!

Becoming Multi-Orgasmic (For Women)

Many psychologists and sexologists write of the importance of self-pleasuring as a way to sexually empower and enrich our lives. Tantra teaches that through self-pleasuring a woman will revitalize her own erotic energy. The practice also teaches us what we like so that we can communicate our desires with our partners. Most Western women have been taught to let the man take the lead, but all women's bodies respond differently so this can oftentimes be a lose-lose situation. Sex therapists commonly describe patients who are hindered by fears of offending their partners by asking for what they really want sexually, and additionally, by fears that advocating for their own sexual satisfaction is not something that a "nice girl" would do. In reality, the woman who can ask for what she wants very often gets it. And, a gentleman appreciates a woman who can communicate her needs and desires.

There is a great deal of research confirming that self-pleasuring has psychological and physical health benefits. Self-pleasuring releases mood-lifting endorphins, is a natural sleep sedative and leads to a stronger pelvic floor for better sex. Through self-pleasuring a woman can build resistance to yeast infections, decrease premenstrual syndrome, and increase blood flow to the pelvis, which leads to decreased menstrual cramping and backaches. Additionally self-pleasuring is an energetic pick-me-up. It can be very empowering, as it allows you to feel better about your body, genitals, and sexual responses. Once you have given yourself the most intense orgasms ever, you can more easily recreate this with your partner. Empower yourself and your partner with an agreement that lets either of you off of the hook when one of you is unavailable, or your moods don't match. Share in self-pleasuring rituals with your partner to get to know how you each like to be touched.

I remember the day I fell in love with my yoni. It took me many years on this planet before I found the willingness to look closely at the beautiful soft pink folds, and explore the inner depths where immense pleasure could be found. It is not that I wasn't masturbating, but

I had limited my self-pleasuring to a quick and dirty act of shame, rather than an open exploration. I was also shutting myself off from accessing my own potent erotic energy. I had let societal belief systems convince me that only my lover should venture into my yoni or give me these types of blissful sensations. I was wrong. Our pleasure is in our own hands, and unless we have examined the many erotic stimulation potentials that provide us with intense delights, we have let down both our current and future lovers, and ourselves. How can you explain to another what gives you pleasure if you do not know yourself?

I would like to invite you to look at any beliefs that could be holding you back from giving yourself the immense pleasure you deserve and were born to receive. Few of us grew up being taught that masturbation is normal, natural, and even healthy. Yet, it is pleasurable, stress-reducing, and empowering. It is your body, and experiencing your body's erotic responses can be just as stimulating as turning on a partner. Taoist teachings advise opening a woman's heart prior to entering her vagina, and I would recommend that you set time aside to explore your body from the most loving compassionate place.

Ladies, you are wired for pleasure, and experiencing the rise of this powerful energy through your own touch is an amazing experience. Using fantasies is a healthy way to experience sexuality in safe ways, but for this journey of self, try bringing full awareness to your explorations. The body is full of bundles of nerve centers and erogenous zones. Discover new ways to touch your body, exploring the many ways you can find pleasure. Explore new realms, delight in the way your body responds to different levels of touch and sensations, finding new delicious ways to turn yourself on and raise your erotic energy. Personal pleasuring playtime will not only enhance your life, it also allows you to return to your lover with valuable knowledge about your body's capacity for ecstasy, and any new enjoyments you've discovered. Share your newfound joys!

Moving Sexual Energy: By learning to move energy from the genitals up the spine and throughout your energy body you will be able to experience your orgasms throughout your entire body, which I refer to as full-body orgasms. You can do this while you are heated, or move your sexual energy while you are cool. Remember that sexual energy is also the creative energy that can fuel your everyday life without genital stimulation. This energy is revitalizing and healing. Just as with men, this is another powerful practice to enhance both your sex life and your everyday life.

Exercise: Lightly cup or touch your vagina and clitoris until you can feel arousal begin. Inhale and as you exhale contract your PC muscle imagining your womb opening like a flower blossoming. Continue to inhale and exhale, experiencing this our sexual energy building. Inhale and sip the energy slowly up your spine. Exhale, relax, but stay with the rising energy mentally. Continue inhaling, tightening and exhaling and relaxing while sipping your sexual energy up your spine. You may need to rock your pelvis back and forth letting your chin bob up and down to help move the energy. Can you feel the orgasmic energy move up your spine? You can direct this energy throughout the body to areas you feel need healing, strengthening or revitalizing.

Most women find this to be an effective way to experience full-body orgasms. Don't be discouraged if it doesn't happen for you right away. Play with it daily and record your experiences in your journal.

Affirmation: I love that my body is multi-orgasmic!

Kundalini

Kundalini is another foundational principle in Tantric traditions that directly relates to tapping into your multi-orgasmic potential, especially as it is often experienced as a deep bridging of spirit and sexuality. According to Joseph Campbell, the Sanskrit word Kundalini means "that which is coiled or spiral in nature" and refers to the spiral patterns of energy found throughout the natural world, from the DNA molecule to the shape of galaxies". Kundalini energy lies coiled at the base of the spine, wrapped three and a half times around the sleeping Shakti. When awakened, Kundalini energy, which is associated with the serpent, rises up through the energy centers along the spine. She is the feminine, the goddess Shakti, who awakens and dances upward through the body. She represents pure consciousness, and through learning to move this energy up through your body, you will learn to tap into the infinite well of orgasmic bliss and connection with divinity (or Universal energy).

Another gift of moving Kundalini-Shakti energy up through the energy centers of the body is its ability to clear energy blocks and heal the pathways in its travel. Kundalini can awaken after intense periods of spiritual practices, such as meditation, yoga or dance, sexual stimulation, fasting, psychedelic drugs, or trauma. It can awaken spontaneously or through transmissions. It is important to stay grounded, balanced, and supported when awakening or moving Kundalini energy. Be gentle, and take extra good care of yourself doing this important period of transformation. Get out into nature, meditate, eat root vegetables, red meat (if you eat it) or whatever it is that makes you feel more grounded. Take warm baths, relax, and give yourself extra love. Talk with your partner or a close friend about what you are experiencing, so you feel supported.

Once awakened, Kundalini energy opens us to greater cosmic consciousness. The Kundalini energy is also considered the primary source for our spiritual development. It was believed that Kundalini awakened serpent power and granted shaman women "enlightened consciousness" and the ability to fly. While some Tantric teachers do not like to utilize Kundalini, others find it imperative to enlightenment.

Kundalini awakens the psychic centers, allowing access to higher consciousness, it can also allow for ecstatic states, unity, and feelings of empowerment. It is also posited to activate dormant areas of the brain. I have introduced the concept of Kundalini as it is an important component of Tantric traditions and relates to the exercises throughout this book. Please also use care when moving energy. Never force energy, instead allow energy to move on its own time schedule. Kundalini is potent energy, so if you have an interest in awakening and moving Kundalini energy, I'd highly recommend studying up on it further before proceeding.

Exercise: Take out your journal and write more on how you feel about Kundalini. Was this a concept with which you were already familiar? Perhaps you have heard of Kundalini yoga. What might appeal or be off putting about Kundalini. Again, please proceed with Kundalini practices by first becoming very informed on the subject.

Affirmation: My inner energy source is potent and powerful.

Section Six: Partnered Play

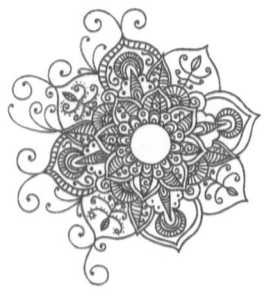

"Real intimacy is a sacred experience."
—John O'Donahue

Shakti and Shiva
(Dance of the Feminine and Masculine)

The union of opposites is an important concept in Tantra. One of the main principles in Tantra relates to the sacred sexual union between Goddess Shakti and the God Shiva. Shakti, or Sakti, as a goddess, is known as the revealer of the truth, the Great Liberator. The masculine energy, often called Shiva, is defined in Tantra as a "limitless, transcending and formless" and the feminine, Shakti, is "the essence within all things" giving form to the material realm. Through the goddess Shakti's sexual union with the god Shiva, the two entities experience wholeness that comprises the Divine. Tantra teaches that humans may embody the energy of these deities in sacred union, allowing for experiences of transcendence and liberation. The belief that worshipping a god or goddess requires that one embody the god or goddess is a common feature in all Tantric traditions.

This does not, however, preclude homosexual couples from being able to utilize these techniques. In Tantra, it is said that we all contain both feminine and masculine qualities and sides to ourselves, and it is important to learn how to bring these into balance. The male and female energies are symbolized by solar and lunar energies in Tantric traditions. The right side of the body is associated with the sun, or solar forces. The left side of the body is considered the feminine side and is associated with the moon, or lunar forces. Masculine solar energy is viewed as being red, fiery, and intellectual. The masculine is the out in the world, projection of our energy. While the feminine is the receptive side. It is our lunar energy, seen as white, cool watery, and intuitive.

Exercise: Getting to know both our masculine and feminine sides is an important key to balancing our own dualistic energy. Close your eyes and focus first on the right side of your body. Notice the hot, mentally powerful masculine side of yourself. How do you project this energy out into the world? What does it feel like? Notice if it feels empowered, or shaky. Then, turn your attention to the left side of your body and feel the cool, connected and nurturing feminine side. Do you trust your instincts and listen to them? Are you able to care and nourish yourself in healthy ways? Pull out your journal and write any observations about how these two parts of yourself feel balanced or out of balance.

Affirmation: My masculine and feminine energies are well balanced.

Intimacy

Your partner is your best friend, and if you are going to share your lives, hopes, dreams and bodies with each other, it makes sense that there be a willingness to share intimately. Sex and intimacy are not the same thing, and shouldn't be confused as such. Intimacy can be a powerful vehicle for healing. When we cultivate loving, intimate relationships, they are more likely to support our growth, understanding, compassion and the way we relate with the outside world. Intimacy requires honesty and trust. Intimacy is fostered by integrity and respect. It is brought about through a willingness to lay oneself bare. This can be a scary thing for many of us. We may have been taught to protect ourselves by not revealing our truest feelings. Being vulnerable isn't often welcomed in our culture. Instead we use emotional armor as protection from perceived judgments. But, sexual ecstasy asks us to drop these defenses. This is a worthwhile endeavor for a multitude of reasons. Once the armor is cast aside, the connection fostered will allow you to step into a far greater level of knowledge, compassion, and understanding about yourself and your partner. This will also ripple out into all of the other relationships in your life. Through your intimacy, you will find a deep and incredibly multi-orgasmic life.

The mask you've used to shield yourself from potential pain is an illusion, dear ones. You may fool yourself into believing that you are stronger because of it, but it only weakens you. Real strength is found in emotional vulnerability and deep sharing with your partner. This takes some practice. It's important for both people to feel protected and safe to let go of the defenses. Go into your sensual space, and connect with your partner. Again, remember that this person is your beloved friend. Assure them that you're trustworthy, and that all sharing stays within the sensual space. Keep good eye contact, listen to each other, and keep physical contact that feels supportive of the process, perhaps holding hands. Open a discussion each taking turns starting by describing a favorite sexual encounter you've shared in the past with your partner (the one you're doing the exercise with. Don't tell them about a favorite experience with an ex!). Next take turns sharing a sexual fantasy you have. Share what you hope to get out of becoming Tantric, and any fears you may have about it.

As you embark on this journey, either alone or with a partner, find ways to share in more play. It is through the playful times, when the everyday worries about finances, work, or other potentially stressful parts of life can be set aside to just have fun that we can connect and build intimacy. If you're pretending that everything is okay, that you're not hurt or that something said or done is not upsetting you, you're closing yourself off from not only the pain, but the ability to experience pleasure and true intimacy, as well. Be honest with yourself about your feelings.

A little warning about Tantra and Intimacy: While using Tantric practices, you will be journeying into higher levels of consciousness. Regular sex opens one to taking on emotional baggage of the person with whom you are intimate. In Tantra, you're taking on a much greater amount of that emotional, mental and spiritual energy. When you walk this path, choose someone with whom you can be truly intimate. This is not to say that you cannot use these techniques to have huge full body orgasms with a stranger. Tantra asks us to connect with ourselves and our partners at a deep, intimate level, and this is best done within a committed partnership.

Exercise: Be honest with yourself about the ways that you may have avoided intimacy in the past. Does true intimacy scare you? Or, are you willing and able to open yourself to your partner?

Affirmation: I trust myself to be open and loving with my partner.

Preparations

As one might expect from such a vast wealth of knowledge, the Tantric texts stress the importance of preparations prior to joining with your partner in sexual embrace and address everything from preparing the environment, the body and the mind.

You have already created the sensual space, so it is time to respect the body by making certain that you are soaped up and clean. Take the time you have to put into it, but make certain that you arrive clean, with your teeth brushed and smelling delightful. If time will allow, take a luxurious bubble bath, alone or with your partner, taking turns bathing each other. Make certain to shave, so stubble doesn't add rashes to your sexy time.

Even clothing recommendations exist, which are quite different from what we may choose here in the Western World. Soft fabrics such as silk or satin are best, with flowing cuts which allow the body to move freely and do not restrict blood flow. Clothing with buttons, buckles, and other less than practical distractions are not advised. Men may wish to find silk pajamas, or nonrestrictive pants with a tied coat over the top. Women may wish to wear a satin or silk negligee, a flowy skirt with see through blouse and no bra, or tie-around clothing, which allows for movement and creates a seductive shape to enhance the female form. I recommend at least giving the silky flowy clothes a try, but wear what makes you feel sexy and helps set the mood for you. Clothing is an extension of one's personality, so if you're happiest in stockings and a garter belt, do so, but do make an effort to wear something that will be arousing for both you and your partner.

Setting the mood mentally is also an important part of connecting with your partner and living a multi-orgasmic life. As you build up toward sexual intimacy with your partner, make sure to communicate and flirt. Connecting mentally with your partner helps establish intimacy and prepares the body for connecting physically. Keep the atmosphere relaxed and comfortable. This isn't the time for dealing with issues. Rather, seductive conversation within a playful mood is wonderful foreplay. Express desires, and offer a couple of genuine, flirtatious compliments to your partner. Share in a light meal and enjoy a glass of wine. Take care not to overindulge though, as you'll need to be clear and focused for later activities.

Exercise: Find a way for you and partner to prepare for love making that is new and exciting for your both. Light candles, set music and bathe each other. Get dressed separately then meet up over a fruit picnic in the back yard, or in front of the fireplace. Feed each other and sip a glass of wine or champagne. Indulge in some sexy flirtation, and tease one another with some light touch. Your preparations will lead to a more sensual, connected evening. Enjoy!

Affirmation: I take pride in showing up fully for my partner.

The Art of the Kiss

I do so love to kiss. I'm not sure there is enough kissing in the world. There are gentle kisses, with tenderness and conscious consideration. Or there are those fiery kisses brought about by the height of erotic arousal. Taoism emphasizes the importance of deep erotic kissing as an art form, and it will take lots of practice, so pucker up, darlings. Remember that while you are exchanging passionate kisses and gazing into your partner's eyes your spirit becomes harmonized.

In Tantra the mouth is a combination of the characteristics of lingam (represented by the tongue) and the yoni (represented by mouth and lips). When the art of the kiss is cultivated, love-making becomes more intense and fulfilling. It is also believed that saliva has a medicinal property that harmonizes the masculine and feminine energies within each of us, and the exchange will help to connect and balance you both. Plus, it's extremely erotic and delicious. Learn to relax the muscles of the face and mouth while kissing, and explore each other's mouths slowly. You can suck the tongue of your partner, which can lead to orgasm. Lick and kiss your beloved's eyelids, forehead, cheeks, ears, and the underside of the chin. It is recommended that partners explore their beloved's mouth for long periods of time.

The upper lip of a woman is considered to be one of the most erotic parts of her body. Many texts, including the Kama Sutra recommends that a man suck and gently nibble on the upper lip of his partner to create an energy circuit that flows to her clitoris. While the man kisses her upper lip, she should play with his lower lip with her tongue and teeth, being careful not to bite too hard. Through visualizing the nerve that runs from her upper lip to her clitoris, the woman will become able to move sexual energy through it. When she is most aroused, the man should suck her upper lip, and she on his lower lip, which will produce heat and heighten sexual arousal for them both, enhancing love-making.

Types of kisses described in Tantra include: the straight kiss, the bent kiss, the turned kiss, the pressed kiss, the clasping kiss and fighting of tongues. In the straight kiss partners are level, directly across from one another, which has an affectionate tenderness. During the bent kiss the beloved's heads are bent toward each other. One or both partners may want to place their hands behind their lover's head for this one. In the turned kiss one beloved has turned to face the other and has held their beloved's chin to kiss them, lending an intensity and passion to the exchange. The pressed kiss is when the lower lip has been pressed with force and the kiss that follows in more intense. In the clasping kiss one of the partners takes both lips between his or her own. The fighting of tongues, or now known as the french kiss, is a deep kiss so that tongues are brought together, circled around one another, and the exchange of vital essences occurs.

Exercise: Spend twenty to thirty minutes kissing your partner. Take your time, playing with each of the types of kisses I describe. How do you each like to be kissed?

What turns you on the most? Really explore each other's lips and mouths. Tell you partner what aroused you most.

Affirmation: Kissing my partner stirs our passion and enhances our vitality.

Reconnecting with Your Partner

A committed relationship with another can be the most powerful and profound source of happiness, support, emotional security and growth. Yet sometimes we neglect our partner and the partnership. We can become preoccupied with career, financial or social standing, or other worldly matters. With our focus on other things, the connection with our beloved can become weakened, and even quite strained. It's a sad truth that we can hurt or neglect those closest to us. We all know that the success of our relationship depends on sustained love and attention. It is also common knowledge that repetition can lead to boredom and stagnation in relationships. It's important to find new ways to connect with and please your partner, in and out of the bedroom.

I know life can get busy, but it's imperative to shift any "I'm too busy" voices to ones that proclaim that your partner is important, and you can and will find a way to make time for each other. Just do it. The relationships in our life are the most important, after all, and your beloved is your best friend. So, make the time, and seize opportunities to play and reconnect with each other in ways that are fun and remind you both of how important you each are to one another. Remember that intention is powerful. If you find that your sweet, loving thoughts have been replaced by daily frustrations, go back to thoughts of the moments when you two were having fun and found pleasure in sharing activities together. Shift negatives to positive. Make gratitude lists just based on giving thanks for things your partner does right. Visualize the happy, healthy life you're going to lead together, and start rekindling those romantic feelings, so you can go forth as the dynamic and satisfied multi-orgasmic couple you desire and deserve to be. This is a powerful, deep practice, which will also give you both more energy for the worldly things that used to get in the way.

If you've gone from one failed relationship to the next, you may carry the burden of fears, wounds, and a sense of insecurity. This does not have to prevent the success of your current relationship. It really can be as simple as choosing to let go of the past stories, and showing up for your current relationship with an open heart. There may be some discomfort, but the efforts made toward creating the loving partnership you want is always worth it. Opening your heart to your partner requires courage and faith. Dare to risk feelings of judgment, rejection, abandonment. Closing off or numbing out in attempts to prevent potentially painful feelings doesn't actually work. Either way you're at risk of experiencing any of these feelings, but they'll be poisoning you internally, which will be reflected in your outer life. It's a continuous cycle, whereby the negative experiences from your past hold all of the power. It's time for healing.

Make a commitment to give your heart openly, honestly, and deeply to your partner. The real hero, goddess, or other archetype you would like to honor in yourself and your partner, is one who is an honest, loving and compassionate being. Relationships are an important part of living in this world. How do you treat others? How much love have you been able to give and receive? What precious moments have you shared with your beloveds? Those are the things that will matter when we near the end of the journey, so make sure they are important to you now. Take a chance, and give your all to your partner, the person by your side.

(Bonus Way: Seven Minutes in Heaven Together): This is a play on the old childhood game of Seven Minutes in Heaven. If you're feeling a deep need to reconnect with your partner, make a commitment to using the practice daily for at least a week or more. Some coupes have found it to be such a powerful practice that they don't want to stop using it.

When you both return from daily activities and reconnect from your respective days, begin by connecting through eye-gazing, kissing, touching and just connecting intimately with one another. This is done wordlessly. For seven minutes, just appreciate the person who is your beloved partner. Remember that connecting with your partner by looking each other in the eyes and kissing brings you into harmony. Try it out and see how it feels and what positive effects it has on your partnership.

Exercise: Exploring energy together can be lots of fun. Go into your sexy space together, light candles, and then lie next to each other, one behind the other, both facing the same direction. Cuddled up like spoons, begin synching your breathing. The person behind should rest their hands over their partners, beginning at the base of the spine, where your energy body begins. Just relax into each other and breathe in unison. Move the hands up so they are resting just beneath the navel, continuing to breathe. Next go up to the just below the ribcage, then up to between the breasts, the throat, the forehead, and the top of your head. There's no need to speak during the practice, just experience the sensations that may arise, such as tingling, a spreading warmth, or even pulsing as the energy rises. Move through the exercise and take your time. You should experience a difference in the quality of connection with your partner almost immediately.

Affirmation: I easily express my love for my partner.

Asking for What You Want (and Having Your Needs Met)

We cannot expect someone to know what we need or expect from them unless we communicate it. Maybe you shy away from conflict, or don't want to trouble or inconvenience your partner. But, one shouldn't let other's needs supersede their own, especially when it becomes the norm. Leave mind reading to the flirty moments when you wink across the room at your partner, and the meaning is obvious. Don't assume your partner can intuit your needs, or you'll probably find them rarely fulfilled. This can lead one down the path of frustration and, inevitably, resentment. That's unnecessary, and there's an easy fix: communication. Remember that your partner is your best friend, and approach communications from that place. While I know it's not always easy, it's up to you to ask for your needs to be met. It's particularly important to be able to articulate these needs in the bedroom.

Are you stuck carrying out roles you've learned? Women are also often taught to acquiesce their pleasure to others. Men are taught to conquer, and that they should know how to please their partners, despite the fact that all women are wired differently from one another. Many people in Western society get their role models for sex from Hollywood and porn- I'm not sure which is worse, or more damaging. Directly or indirectly, a woman learns that men are supposed to know more about how to please her than she does, even though its her own body. But, guys learn what pleases a woman when they try something and it works. This rarely carries over to a possible next partner, because women are all different. Worse yet, men are considered to be the aggressors, the ones who instigate the act of sex, and women are the passive receivers, even considered by some to be prey. Ack! Is it any wonder that we're all messed up when it comes to sexuality?

Many women experience feelings of frustration around their unfulfilled sex lives. As long as one's sexuality is in the hands of another person, there will be no empowerment or ability to step into a multi-orgasmic and sexually fulfilled life. The days of "Did you come yet, honey?" are now over. It's time to learn how to ask for what you really want from your partner, and have those needs met. Everyone has personal preferences about how they like to be touched and caressed. Life is short, and your pleasure is essential. Push past barriers of shame, guilt, and embarrassment to ask for your desires to be met.

In Tantra, both partners are equal, and communication is essential and required. The rush to a goal of joint orgasm is being thrown out. Goodbye outdated models of double standard which doesn't work for most of us. For this exercise, both parties will set aside the end goal, and just let pleasure be the guide. Approach your partner when he/she is open and receptive, not tired, and distracted. Request a play date. Finding enjoyment from your sexuality unfolds when exploration and play meet in conscious union. Pretend you don't know your partner's body, and slowly adventure anew. Cultivate pleasure. Be respectful. It is always your responsibility to express your likes and dislikes to your partner.

The best way to express what you want and need is through subtle cues. Let your partner touch, caress, and gently guide his/her hands where you'd like them to go. Make encouraging noises. Saying, "yes", and "more please" are good clues. Remember that it's also your responsibility to say no if there's something you don't like or doesn't feel good. It's good to set some ground rules prior to play, if you know that certain things will upset you or make you uncomfortable. You don't need to give lengthy explanations for what you don't like. It's important not to make demands, either. "Honey, I love it when you—" or "It really turns me on when you—" are sufficient, and will be received better when expressed in appreciative, flirty and caring ways. Play with the exercises I detailed earlier designed for partnered exploration. Nothing is forbidden in Tantra. Let go of stigma around certain activities, and be willing to go with what feels good. What gives you both the most pleasure. Play like innocent children, as it was intended.

Exercise: Move through a fear or comfort zone by making a new request from your partner. What have you always wanted to try? Or, how could you communicate with your partner about something you'd like them to do more of that would give you great pleasure? Time to get vocal and ask to have your needs met. Make certain the appropriate atmosphere has been set for your request. How can you reciprocate and give something to your partner that would give him/her pleasure in return?

Affirmation: I love myself enough to openly and respectfully express my needs to my partner.

Keep Experimenting

Life offers us many opportunities to experiment. Sexuality is no different. There is no one way to please everybody and even the same body will need different types of touch and pleasure-giving techniques at different times. Continue to be brave in your playful explorations. Experimenting with different experiences is what makes life so interesting.

The body's potential for pleasure is incredibly vast, and stepping into its fullest potential takes time and practice. Hopefully you're already experiencing some of these marvelous multi-orgasmic possibilities through the use of the techniques in this book. The more we embrace our inherent sexuality, the greater it can nourish and sustain us. Through continual experimentation and play, you can find even greater ways to live a satisfying, multi-orgasmic life. You deserve to live from a place of your personal power and in connection with your creative energy.

It is my hope that you will take what you've learned here and continue to explore what brings more pleasure into your life. Continue to find new ways that make you happy and that enrich your multi-orgasmic potentials. I've offered many tools in this book, which take time to incorporate. You will probably want to refer back to remind yourself of techniques. Give yourself the gift of deepening your practice by yourself and with your partner.

Sexual energy is creative. The more ways you implement pleasuring techniques into your life, the happier you'll feel and the more your life will have an ease and flow. Life can continually blossom into deeper levels of creativity. Let life exceed your expectations. Find the rhythms that allow for your most vibrant, juicy life expressions. Allow relationships to be their most loving, harmonious and at their best. How can you embrace and tap into the potent powerful source within you at deeper levels? What adventures are you willing to embark upon to allow your highest potential to be realized? Where can your multi-orgasmic life take you now?

Exercise: Which techniques have you found to be most helpful? What new practices can you implement into your life? Keep experimenting; life is meant to be fun!

Affirmation: I enjoy finding the best way to fulfill my highest life potentials.

About the Author

Antonia Hall is an author, self-improvement expert, spiritual teacher, artist and longtime blogger. She is committed to helping people bring more pleasure into their lives and is known as an inspirational catalyst for positive living. Her teachings and writings offer practical guidance on utilizing our inherent sexuality to enrich our everyday lives. Antonia has a passion for helping people live to their greatest potential.

Ms. Hall graduated cum laude from Dominican University in Marin County, where she received a B.A. in Psychology. She received her M.A. at the Institute of Transpersonal Psychology. While she is based in Beverly Hills, California, Antonia is a worldwide traveler who has spent many years living abroad in the Netherlands, France, Mexico, and Costa Rica. She is also an artist and nature enthusiast who devotes time to protecting the environment and promoting green living.

Learn more about Antonia at AntoniaHall.com

www.ingramcontent.com/pod-product-compliance
Lightning Source LLC
Chambersburg PA
CBHW020616300426
44113CB00007B/667